# MANAGED CARE

*Made in America*

Arnold Birenbaum

PRAEGER

Westport, Connecticut
London

**Library of Congress Cataloging-in-Publication Data**

Birenbaum, Arnold.
    Managed care : made in America / Arnold Birenbaum.
        p.    cm.
    Includes bibliographical references and index.
    ISBN 0–275–95916–3 (alk. paper)
    1. Managed care plans (Medical care)—United States.   I. Title.
RA413.5.U5B495   1997
362.1'04258'0973—dc21        97–5578

British Library Cataloguing in Publication Data is available.

Library of Congress Catalog Card Number: 97–5578
ISBN: 0–275–95916–3

First published in 1997

Praeger Publishers, 88 Post Road West, Westport, CT 06881
An imprint of Greenwood Publishing Group, Inc.

Printed in the United States of America

The paper used in this book complies with the
Permanent Paper Standard issued by the National
Information Standards Organization (Z39.48–1984).

10 9 8 7 6 5 4 3 2 1

# Contents

# Preface

In the last week of preparation before I submitted the manuscript for this book to the publisher, a major opinion piece appeared in the *New England Journal of Medicine* (Bodenheimer, 1996) on the backlash against managed care, subtitled, "Righteous or Reactionary?" The article called for a return to the prepaid-group practice model of the earliest health maintenance organizations (HMOs), free of the profit motive. No sooner had I read this powerful article then a full-page book review of *Wall Street Journal* reporter George Anders's *Health Against Wealth: HMOs and the Breakdown of Medical Trust*, a jeremiad on how cost-driven managed care corporations are damaging the quality of health care in the United States, appeared in the book review of my hometown paper (Samuelson, 1996). In addition, a triptych of a cartoon take-off on the famous Harry and Louise commercials that helped defeat the Clinton reforms for health care, by Gary Hallgren, complete with voice over and an anxious Louise, headed the lead article of the *New York Times Week in Review* (Toner, 1996). Finally, in the same newspaper, physicians in a front-page article expressed worry about how reduced fees to doctors by HMOs will reduce the quality of patient care (Rosenthal, 1996).

Little did I know in 1994 when I wrote a new chapter—"The Growth of Managed Care and the Backlash"—for the revised and updated edition of my book *Putting Health Care on the National Agenda* (1995) that I would be a trend setter. While I feel I am in good company, I set out in 1996 to write a book based on the best health-services research and policy analysis available on managed care. To keep up with the steady progress toward managed care, and the reaction to it, deserves systematic treatment of the topic. It should also be written in a way that consumers and providers, as well as payers, can grasp the essentials of what is good about managed care and what needs to be fixed.

Managed care and HMOs got their start in the United States. For years the medical establishment marginalized HMOs, and managed care was seen as encroaching on the physician's autonomy. Increasing inflation in health care has made what was once unattractive very appealing. HMOs are now not only sources of care but also corporations in which to invest. This new, complex version of American health-care delivery integrates services and brings together providers who were previously connected in only patchwork ways. This very cohesiveness makes services better for the consumer and diminishes consumer and provider control. Making this relationship less trustworthy is the shadowy figure of the third-party payer who, by exercising control, attempts to keep costs down. As a result, many consumer advocates are once again crying out, *caveat emptor*—let the buyer beware!

This response is understandable. We are in the middle of a vast reconstruction of the American health-care system. Whether this process will yield benefits for ordinary Americans depends on who shapes its future and for what end. The story I tell in these pages began before the Clinton Health Care Task Force was called into being in 1993. It grew while Task Force experts worked frantically in their "delivery room" in the Executive Office Building and other venues in the capital.

The spate of cartoons in our newspapers and magazines which has accompanied the growth of managed care speak to what the distinguished sociologist Robert K. Merton called "sociological ambivalence"—a conflicted feeling that patients have today about physicians who are now subject to an external control rather than professional standards and peer review. At bottom, it is about social change. It is about having the doctor contracting with an HMO and being subject to its rules; about the limited access to specialty care; and about the frugal use of hospital admissions and stays.

Patients may feel their physicians are trustworthy but do not trust the organizations they work for. David Mechanic and Mark Schlesinger captured the meaning of this concept in their 1996 article on social trust in health-care organizations. They argued that "the success of medical care depends most importantly on patients' trust that their physicians are competent, take appropriate responsibility and control, and give their patients' welfare the highest priority" (p. 1693). Is that trust compromised when the very mechanisms of managed care—such as utilization review, restrictions on choice, gatekeeping, and financial incentives to limit care—pressure physicians into not always acting in the patient's best interest?

HMOs were once viewed as part of the solution to our health-care crisis. The continuous growth of HMOs during the 1980s encouraged the policy experts (also known as wonks) assembled by the first Clinton administration to seek to correct what had become a difficult situation. When employers did not provide group coverage, many middle-class Americans could not afford an individual insurance policy for their families; some did not have access to group coverage because they were self-employed, small entrepreneurs with limited incomes; and there were people with long-term serious preexisting conditions who were denied coverage through employment, or who simply could not afford the extremely expensive risk-adjusted policies available in the marketplace.

The first Clinton administration took on a daunting task. The failure of health-care reform in 1994 almost cost President Clinton a second term, and it helped elect a 104th Congress dominated by an antigovernment opposition. These political events form the backdrop for the even more rapid rise of the HMOs in the United States in the current decade.

To their credit, the Clintons wanted to create comprehensive reform that would simultaneously keep down the cost of care while covering the entire population. These goals required the creation of a regional actuarial structure for insurance coverage and service delivery—large risk pools and purchasing alliances. Today we see the seeds of that evolution in the integration of health services and employers creating buying cooperatives.

In the public's eyes, proposed changes by the Task Force were not friendly but only represented bureaucracy. By virtue of the campaign against the Clinton plan, private bureaucracy was ignored and only the government was seen as the enemy. This maximum misunderstanding was captured best in an incident recounted by Senator John B. Breaux of Louisiana. A sweet older woman buttonholed him at an airport, with the plea, "Please, Senator, don't let the government take away my Medicare."

With the death of health-care reform in September 1994, even more employers interested in saving on fringe benefits turned to managed care features in their health plans and HMOs, or even dropped group coverage. Employees, unless they worked in the public sector, were offered fewer choices. The number of uninsured jumped from 37 to 41 million. The states sought benefit waivers from the Health Care Financing Administration so that they could convert to capitated managed care and in some instances extend Medicaid benefits to a greater proportion of the population living in poverty. Market forces were turned loose, and physicians were now anxious to sign on to many managed care plans or join HMOs in order to maintain their incomes. The irony is that between 1994 and 1996, price-sensitive consumers in the millions joined the very HMOs which in 1993–1994 they said would keep them from maintaining their valued relationships with their family physicians.

By 1996, there were 60 million members of HMOs. Employers spearheaded this drive, receiving and using various financial incentives. Conducted in 1993, a national survey of almost 2000 employers found that over half were in managed care plans, up from 29 percent in a similar polling in 1988. By 1995, three-quarters of U.S. workers with health insurance were, in one form or another, part of managed care coverage.

Given the failure of wholesale reform and the trends toward managed care, the pundits described incrementalism not only as the right way to go in health-care reform but also the American way. With the 1996 reelection of the most resilient president since Grover Cleveland and the collective focus on trimming the safety net and entitlements, government will likely do little to create universal coverage beyond extending Medicaid coverage to all children from low- and moderate-income families under the age of 18. Such an umbrella would create a greater opportunity for a healthy start for children in near-poverty families and allow their parents to use their limited purchasing power to put food on the table and find affordable housing. It is hard to say no to such a political move—even Newt Gingrich might support it—and it is probably a policy substitute for helping to increase the purchasing power of moderate- and low-income families. During the runup to the 1996 presidential election, those close to the secretary of Health and Human Services hinted that covering children would be a cost-effective measure that would help families with their daily problems. This idea has caught on with the voters.

Supporters of President Clinton's bid for a second term did not help elect a Democratic Congress. However, in his new-found role of the "fixer," or perhaps "the People's Tribune," the president will keep a close eye on the quality of health care in the transition to managed care through a national commission, to become active in 1997. In addition, efforts will probably be made to correct some of the perceived excesses of managed care that are related to limits on access to hospital care (e.g., one day postpartum stays), to produce contracts that include rules against disclosure about financial incentives imposed on physicians, and to provide medical advice on services unavailable by policy at an HMO.

The rationale for these concerns about managed care is the subject of this book. "What is managed care?," the theme of Chapter 1, attempts to locate the origins of HMOs. The concept of managed care introduces explicit rationing. Some of this rationing functions through service substitution to offset other costs. For example, HMOs encourage patients to have regular examinations conducted by primary care providers, to learn to avoid risky habits, and to help detect diseases that can be treated early and inexpensively. Providers are often compensated through capitation to encourage them to conduct regular examinations, immunize children, and avoid specialty care.

Employers as purchasers of health care started looking for good buys in the marketplace when inflation drove up the cost of benefit packages. They sought defined costs for health plans, which are now viewed as commodities with a single fixed price, much like a ton of coal. All the measures they introduced over the past 20 years involved asserting greater control over the services that would be covered. And once business leaders, as discussed in Chapter 2, were able to control their own health-care costs, they lost interest in national reform.

Employers were aided by a health-care delivery system with excessive capacity, making it possible for HMOs to drive hard bargains with providers. Hospitals with unfilled beds and doctors looking to receive more referrals willingly came to terms with the HMOs and other managed care plans. With hospitals it meant running with fewer staff; with physicians, it meant giving up a great deal of autonomy in their practice.

Chapter 3 deals with the extension of managed care to Medicaid recipients. The policy experts' concern about whether managed care is appropriate for the disproportionate number of people with chronic illnesses and disabilities who are covered by Medicaid is discussed. Changing the health-care environment for the poor has both disrupted and reduced services and even resulted in fraudulent activities by providers in several states. However, health-services research has identified some greater continuity of care than in fee-for-service Medicaid, with greater emphasis on prevention than was found in the past among providers serving the population eligible for Medicaid. Chapter 3 asks whether long-term care could work under capitation.

Are HMO members getting good medical care, and are they being kept as well as their fellow Americans with indemnity insurance? As shown in Chapter 4, HMOs do well in early detection, prevention, and wellness education for enrollees. But what about referrals for specialty care, particularly expensive surgical procedures? After all, not electing to do the bypass operation helps preserve the HMO's financial resources as a business.

Prevention is a forward-looking way of providing services, but what are the consequences of this new approach for people with serious chronic illnesses and disabilities? Since they are heavy users of specialty care, a resource that is rationed in this delivery system, we need to find out how well managed care handles the health needs of this sector of the population. Access under managed care may not be as convenient today as it was in the past. Now HMOs sign up only one provider for such a service, and that specialty program may not be so easy to join. Contracts for highly rare and specialized services may be negotiated at locales that are quite distant from the enrollees' residences, forcing them to disrupt their lives in order to receive care under the contract.

How HMOs attempt to assure quality for their customers is the subject of Chapter 5. Good marketing requires information about how well a health plan does and with what kinds of patients. If an HMO is going to make money, it has to attract and hold on to subscribers as well as efficiently use resources. Given the emphasis on the price that the employer/purchasers pay for a health plan for employees, it is important to discuss the industry's collective efforts to accredit plans, to develop measures of quality, and to create "report cards" that the consumers can directly understand.

To understand what goes into creating quality assurance, it is necessary to spell out some major concepts. Structure involves the selection and accreditation of physicians. Measures of performance or process also occur, consisting of simple or detailed examinations of standardized kinds of activities that will assure the prevention of disease, such as immunizations or testing on a regular basis for the presence of disease, for example, doing a Pap smear. In addition, there are ways to determine whether good care is delivered when disease is present. Perhaps the best measure of quality is the result of an intervention. These are called "outcomes" and refer to making people well enough for them to pursue their major life activities. Along these lines, some questions are raised as to whether enough attention is devoted to the plans' management of serious chronic illness and to the resultant outcomes.

Is the health-care system getting meaner as well as leaner? This question is answered in Chapter 6, which synthesizes our knowledge of consumer satisfaction. In almost all surveys that compare HMO members with individuals who have old-fashioned health insurance coverage, the HMO members are less satisfied. In addition, consumers in "gatekeeper" free preferred provider organizations (PPOs) also are more satisfied than HMO members, mainly because their network provides a choice of physicians and unrestricted access to specialists.

Consumer satisfaction surveys point to the high turnover rate of both providers and plan members. The provider problem puts the consumer at a disadvantage because continuity of care is interrupted. High consumer turnover, whether because of dissatisfaction with services or because the employer changes plans, also eliminates the advantage of provider continuity through contact that a regular source of care could provide. In addition, anecdotal evidence from people's experiences with complex medical disorders shows that they had a great deal of difficulty with the health plans in gaining reasonable access to expensive services. Finally, Chapter 6 reviews the kinds of survey instruments being developed to compare plans.

By the end of the 1980s, employers and private insurers were turning to cost management companies to review the performance of physicians submitting claims. Professional autonomy and managed care, the subject of Chapter 7, did not mesh well. By the end of the decade, more than 60 percent of health plans were using preadmission review, and about half were using concurrent review. More recently, physician profiling and clinical practice guidelines were also being utilized to micromanage physicians, further calling into question their prized professional autonomy.

Interestingly, many large medical groups can provide all the services found in HMOs and willingly take on the other characteristics of capitated medical systems, including assumption of financial risk. Despite some legal restrictions imposed by antitrust laws, the doctor-owned HMO is coming on line. Some HMO organizational practices that have been called harmful to patients (such as financial incentives to primary-care physicians for keeping down costs through limiting hospital admissions, referrals to specialists, and reduced diagnostic testing) are found in these new doctor-owned plans as well as in other HMOs.

As mentioned at the beginning of this Preface, the managed care revolution has left many consumers and professionals feeling that they need protection from naked market forces. In the words of C. Wright Mills, we are discovering once again how private troubles become transformed into public issues. This kind of struggle, one that pits the American Medical Association and various consumer advocacy groups on one side, and the American Association of Health Plans, the national lobby for the HMOs, on the other, continues on the state and federal level.

Chapter 8 discusses the extent to which states have moved through law to eliminate the causes of consumer and provider complaints. These regulations have begun to shape the discussion of what kind of health-care system we will have because they have attempted to reconnect providers and consumers directly, eliminating or restricting the interest of the HMO as the dominant and controlling player in the health-care game.

The way HMOs operate is the subject of Chapter 9. HMOs are highly integrated organizations. Management seeks to avoid inefficiencies such as duplication of service and a kind of decision making that puts it at the point-of-care so that patients can get exactly what they need and no more. A new culture of rationing is also present: HMO management encourages providers to learn how to work within a system that downplays heroic intervention, an oft-noted attribute of American physicians acquired during medical education and training. In HMO medicine, providers need to make good decisions, based on the limited resources they have available, and recently acquired knowledge of how to achieve the best outcomes.

Marketing and sales techniques are also important. How HMOs sell their services to both benefits officers of corporations, employees with families, and Medicare-eligible individuals is discussed. The increasing market share of an HMO may be achieved by substantial capital investment, making it possible to proffer low-cost contracts with employers while also inducing providers to sign up. Being able to sustain losses may reduce the number of competitors in a particular metropolitan region, leading to the development of "mature markets" with fewer plans.

The many unresolved issues related to consumer choice and provider rights are discussed in Chapter 10. The shift to managed care is one of a number of social changes that has left many Americans anxious about whether hard work and playing by the rules will provide them with the financial security to raise a family, develop their personal interests, share a life with a partner, participate in community life, or do any of a thousand other worthwhile endeavors.

Access to health care makes some of the above changes possible. A health plan and the providers who work in them are seen as reliable if there is a sense that the medical decision is made according to medical criteria. Can health care work if doctors have to choose between obligations to patients and obligations to employer or payer for services?

Furthermore, when a plan promises to provide all the medical care required, then even if patients develop conditions that are unfamiliar to HMO doctors, the HMO still has to make state-of-the-art medical care available. Consumers need to know whether they are getting the best care available. Patients cannot make a clear decision when physicians restrict or withhold information. A widely needed service such as health care can be made available to all and yet be subject to controls that protect both consumers and providers. Accordingly, a bill of rights should be created for enrollees and their doctors.

A number of societal issues remain to be resolved. How can our health-care system continue to reward the pursuit of excellence when it comes to medical practice and therefore encourage physicians and surgeons to gain experience working with the most difficult cases when the new managed care reward system is organized around risk avoidance? Many medical tasks clearly involve the continuous rebuilding of its infrastructure through the creation of new knowledge and the renewal of human capital by exposing trainees and residents to dealing with the most difficult cases. In addition, these practical citadels of twentieth-century health care have often been the sources of charity care for those without insurance, including the homeless, undocumented aliens or the near-poor who cannot qualify for Medicaid.

The support of these activities was part of the "connective tissue" that held American society together. The funding came largely from indemnity insurance payments that generated a surplus for these nonprofit corporations to help provide for the commonweal.

Academic medical centers (AMCs) are beginning to feel that managed care is interfering with their public mission. Valuable hours of teaching in AMCs were donated or *pro bono* labor in the past. AMCs have serious concerns as to how to make up for the shortfall in mentoring that once was assumed to come with the territory when a doctor received admitting privileges to a hospital. A similar issue is raised in Chapter 10 concerning clinical research.

Finally, as our hospitals become tied into contracts with HMOs for inpatient care, less surplus will be left in their budgets to provide charity care for the uninsured and so they will have less interest in caring for the uninsured. In addition, the public health functions and coordinative tasks once assumed by hospitals and physicians may not get performed without a new social compact. What the Health Security Act tried to do was to take these problems into account and preserve the best while extending quality care to all. We now turn to why this did not happen.

## REFERENCES

Bodenheimer, T. 1996. "The HMO backlash—Righteous or reactionary?" *New England Journal of Medicine* 335 (November 25): 1601–1604.

Mechanic, D., and Schlesinger, M. 1996. "The impact of managed care on patients' trust in medical care and their physicians." *Journal of the American Medical Association* 275 (June 5): 1693–1697.

Rosenthal, E. 1996. "Reduced H.M.O. fees cause concern about patient care." *New York Times* (November 25): Al.

Samuelson, R. J. 1996. "Mismanaged care: The flight to H.M.O.s, a reporter argues, is bad for patients and bad for medicine." Review of *Health Against Wealth: HMOs and the Breakdown of Medical Trust* (Boston: Houghton Mifflin), *New York Times Book Review* (November 24): 13.

Toner, R. 1996. "Health cares: Harry and Louise were right, sort of." *New York Times* (November 24): Section 4, 1.

# Introduction: Retrenchment and the Remaking of the Health-Care System

> I think that if you look at the health-care issue, I think that I over-estimated the extent to which a person elected with a minority of the votes in an environment that was complex, to say the least, could make—could achieve in a sweeping overhaul of the health-care system when no previous President had been able to do it for decades and decades, and against the enormous amount of organizational effort and funding that was spent to convince the American people of something that was not accurate—namely, that we wanted to have the Government take over the health-care system or that we wanted to regulate it with a cumbersome bureaucracy—neither of which was true, but I think they believed that. And I think people said, "Hey, that's not the kind of change we want."
> —Bill Clinton, President of the United States of America
> (Wines and Pear, 1996)

In 1992, as they do every four years, Americans elected someone who gave them a sense of the future. Bill Clinton had a mandate to improve the lot of the middle class in America, an amorphous cohort that included people near poverty and the denizens of the affluent suburbs. Clinton promised to do something for the people who worked hard, paid their taxes, followed the rules, and hoped for a better life for their children. He was tuned into how difficult life could be in America. The economy was going through some deep transitions related to the exporting of manufacturing as well as information processing jobs. For American workers, real wages were not rising and the purchasing power of the average family was stagnant.

Some of the problems of everyday life related to the high cost of health care: the fear of falling if you lost insurance or changed jobs, and what would happen if you experienced a catastrophic illness. For those who did not have insurance because it was too expensive, Americans had anxieties about how to pay for more than an occasional visit to an Emergency Department; or if hospitalized, about whether they would get the same medical care and diagnostic testing as everybody else.

With the Clinton victory, expectations were raised that finally the United States would join the rest of the industrialized world and have universal coverage. The momentum was certainly there, given the public opinion polls and the complaints of the captains of industry in the United States about how high health-care costs were making them non-competitive in the world market. It seemed like a good bet that a major proposal would create more security for families and answer some of the concerns of the manufacturing sector about international competition. So why did we not have health-care reform in America following the election of the "man from Hope?"

While Clinton generated belief that he understood these problems, he was not moving with a tidal wave calling for a remedy for our social ills. There was no common conscience or intensely and widely shared belief that took note that we were in a period of tremendous difficulty that only a major reform could correct. This was not a unified country, as it had been during the hard times of the Great Depression, when "New Dealer" Franklin Delano Roosevelt created Social Security for the old and a safety net for children, giving many Americans a sense of security.

There was also no sense that we needed to complete the New Deal during these far more prosperous times. It is not an historical contradiction to suggest that sometimes social change occurred during good times in America, particularly when a majoritarian force was propelling reform forward. The 1960s was a time of social turmoil, but it combined with great discretionary income for the federal government, an overwhelmingly liberal Congress, and strong sentiments about the common good that made Medicare and Medicaid realities. Rolling into health-care reform today would be extremely difficult since many interest groups were perfectly happy with things as they were. The upper middle class had coverage, although increasingly they were paying more for health care out-of-pocket than in the past. While public sentiment favored universal coverage, few wanted to make significant sacrifices to make it a reality.

A key element missing in planning health-care reform was the recognition of how many powerful stakeholders there were in the contemporary health-care system as well as how expensive it would be to bring an additional 37 million uninsured into it. Moreover, the advocates of change were not supported by a united Democratic party on a mission to maintain quality care at reasonable cost for everybody. The Democratic party in 1993 was not the party of 1933 or even 1963. It did not convey a single image, and it did not back a single plan for health-care reform. Everyone in the party called for change, but the public didn't see change as its friend.

## A PRESIDENT WITH GRAND AMBITIONS

William Jefferson Clinton won a three-way race in 1992 with the out-of-touch Gulf War hero, George Bush, and the feisty, deficit-fighting H. Ross Perot, ultimately the winner of a surprising 19 percent of the popular vote. The federal deficit dictated strategy for the former governor of Arkansas in 1993, as it will for all future presidents at least to the end of the twenty-first century. After all, a 4 trillion dollar debt doesn't disappear overnight. The interest on the debt alone would eat up a great deal of the annual federal budget. Still, the Clinton administration wanted to provide some economic stimulation in a country that had experienced a moderate recession during George Bush's presidency. The president also wanted to solidify the gains of the Democratic party with what were known as "Reagan Democrats," the lower-middle-class whites who came back to the fold to support his candidacy.

The newly elected president won only 43 percent of the popular vote and needed to provide some economic relief to the middle class that supported him without lowering taxes. The continued ballooning of the federal budget deficit kept interest rates high, and cutting the deficit required a tax increase for the rich as well as an increase in the gasoline tax as sources of revenues. Some targeted tax relief was also included in this package to protect the subaffluent members of the workforce from suffering further decline in their purchasing power. The 1993 budget, which the Democrats barely passed, was responsible for a substantial reduction in interest rates in subsequent years and brought the federal deficit down simply because the government paid less for money and borrowed less to pay its bills. When the government did not seek to borrow money, the market was more of a buyer's market and interest rates also fell for businesses and consumer borrowers. With lower long-term interest rates, many first-time buyers were able to become home owners, and still more mortgage holders were able to refinance and lock-in lower interest rates for the next 15 or 25 years. In addition, lower short-term rates made it easier for businesses to expand and consumers to pay back their credit card debt. In turn, easy credit helped to create jobs.

The cost of Medicare and Medicaid has also contributed to federal deficits, far more than what has been expended on welfare entitlements in the United States. Acting on these elements in the federal budget while creating some form of coverage for the uninsured made sense to the policy-oriented Clinton. The president hoped that the savings on these programs would also be applied to deficit reduction. Many experts believed that the health-care system had highly inflated costs and that a great deal of waste could be squeezed out by lowering payments to providers of services (i.e., mainly hospitals and physicians). Comprehensive change in the delivery system was required to bring the public and the private share of health-care expenditures in line with those of other nations that had similar characteristics and were national economic competitors.

Part of the newly elected baby-boomer's first year in office was an education in the difficulties of both pleasing the populace and creating social change. Clinton wanted to take everything on at once, in the hopes of being able to point to a vibrant economy when he sought re-election in 1996. The president's economic advisors quickly disabused him of the notion that any savings achieved through health-care reform could both be applied against the federal deficit and extend universal health-care coverage (Woodward, 1994: 87). Moreover, his policy advisory team was hopelessly naive in believing that enabling legislation to extend coverage could be passed in a relatively short period of time.

In essence, despite Clinton's commitment to create financing and organizational reform in the health-care arena in 1993, he showed little comprehension of the magnitude of the task. The White House priority earlier that year was an economic stimulus package that could generate 8 million jobs in four years. Clinton sacrificed the package in order to win over the fiscal conservatives in his own party. This course, along with increases in taxes, proved to investment bankers and bond houses alike that the president meant business when he pledged to shrink the federal deficit. With greater investment, the economy started to grow, and 10 million new jobs were created in the next four years—without a targeted growth or stimulus package.

Given the president's fiscal course, the rationale of his political strategy was to help working-class and lower-middle-class citizens reduce their expenses while achieving greater security. His strategy would also have long-term consequences in reducing the share of the gross domestic product (GDP) that was going to pay for health care in the United States. In 1997, at 15 percent of GDP, by the end of the millennium it would easily reach 16 percent, a proportion unmatched in any other country in the world. The need for change that would set the country on the right course fiscally through debt reduction was also evident with regard to health care. Health-care reform was perhaps the best option to help the middle class, given that a tax break was not possible. Furthermore, a stimulus package would not convince the bond market and the Federal Reserve that the administration was seeking to get its house in order.

Health-care reform would substitute for the plans to give a break to those who worked hard and paid their taxes. As a result, the White House's number two priority—health-care reform—now became number one. Creating reform was treated with great seriousness, kicked off by the president's brilliant speech to a joint session of Congress in September 1993. While offering nothing specific in this address, Clinton revealed his skills as an orator and showman as well as a substantial policy analyst. His health-care proposal proffered a health security card to the nation, which would be similar to a Social Security card in importance but look not unlike a credit card. It would treat health care as an entitlement for all. The health-care system behind that card would become accessible to everyone; it would be affordable to every citizen, and it would maintain quality. Furthermore, the loss of a job would not mean the loss of benefits. Quality care would be available to everyone. Waste and inefficiency would disappear through competition between health plans.

With a great deal of public support and some consternation among stakeholders who were left out, the Clinton team in the spring of 1993 called together a Task Force of health and medical experts to create a blueprint for change, which would eventually be presented to the country in the form of a proposed Health Security Act. Hundreds of program directors, professors, and policy analysts took leaves of absence from their places of employment, becoming temporary government employees. Many officials of the Department of Health and Human Services were transferred to the Task Force. Thousands of hours of presentations, debate, drafting, revising, editing, and rewriting into legislative language took place over a period of nine months. Mobilization resembled planning to fight a war on several fronts.

The actual plan was never presented to the public in a clear and simple manner, and gradually, the public began to see it as big government running amok. Many elements of this package were already part of the health-care landscape in one state or another, or part of a nationally organized health maintenance organization, but some of the media, the public, and some lobbies treated it as if it were coming off a drawing board and had never been tried or tested. In the end, it failed to become legislation, even in a stripped-down form. Since educating the public never really took place, the many attacks on the Health Security Act were never answered. No section of the proposed legislation ever got beyond the House and Senate Committees to which they were assigned to reach the floor of either body.

Later, several efforts were made to transform some of the Health

Security Act into legislation that would be less restrictive of insurance companies and HMOs by dropping some of the national review features on expenditures and quality assurance. Congressional Democrats, however, could never get a critical mass behind a single proposal, and most Republicans decided to follow the Republican advisor William Crystal's strategy of denying the president *any* kind of accomplishment that he could use to run on for a second term. Senate Minority Leader Bob Dole had already warned the president that he could not expect to receive any cooperation or support from the Republicans in Congress. The Republicans, aware that they would be censured by their party for putting forth any health proposals, generally refrained from doing anything, even when they believed in bipartisan efforts.

The president's allies in Congress finally gave up. The most apt comment on the health-care fiasco came from former Republican congressman Fred Grandy. The operating policy in Congress in 1994, he said, was "Don't just do something, stand there!" This Iowan, an actor from the sitcom "Love Boat," had a fine ear for what lay behind the legislators' reticence to say that they were against health-care reform. Grandy presents many insightful insider descriptions of how the various House committees operated during those final days of proposed health-care reform (1995: 135–140).

The failure of health-care reform in 1994 provides only the backdrop for the rise of health maintenance organizations (HMOs) in the United States. HMOs were coming on line even with reform since they were the backbone of the Health Security Act. This uniquely American form of service delivery has been in existence since the Great Depression; even then it was a way for employers to keep their insurance costs down. The HMOs' continuous growth during the 1980s encouraged the policy wonks assembled by the new Clinton administration to seek universal health care. Specifically, they wanted to correct what had become a difficult situation even for many middle-class Americans who could not afford an individual insurance policy for their families, who did not have access to group coverage at work, who were self-employed small entrepreneurs with limited incomes, who because of long-term preexisting conditions were denied coverage at work, or who could not afford the extremely expensive rate-adjusted policies available in the marketplace. The Clintons wanted to create comprehensive reform that would keep down the cost of care while covering the entire population. These goals required the creation of large community-based risk pools and purchasing alliances on a regional basis.

1. The campaign for reform was low on conflict and high on good will. The Clinton game plan to transform his blueprint into legislation required that no one be left out of the health-care process. In this politics of inclusion, all insurance companies, health maintenance organ-

izations, and managed care organizations had to be factored into any scheme. Everyone had to know "What's in it for Me" so that they would be willing to trade, bargain, and agree to accept half a loaf. No attempt was made to explain that health care for everyone at a reasonable price could not work based on the current financing system.

The architects of the plan used employer-based contributions and deductions to pay for reform and managed competition to hold costs down. As a result, it was impossible to present a simple and stream-lined plan. They avoided the single-payer option which would have meant great autonomy for physicians and would have freed employers from the obligation of paying for their employees' health care. This Canadian-style reform depends strictly on public financing, and choosing it would have meant eliminating the strictly indemnity insurance companies as well as the managed care plans from the health insurance marketplace.

The small indemnity insurance companies, as well as some of the larger ones like Golden Rule, would be the big losers, for the Clinton health-care reform package depended on HMOs for delivery of services. A sizable chunk of the industry had already established employer-friendly managed care plans in order to hold on to their market share. The straight indemnity industry was not sufficiently capitalized to make the shift to managed care as had occurred among large companies like Prudential, Aetna, Metropolitan Life, Travelers, and Cigna. Still, a public insurance program was never seriously considered because it would mean a tough fight with these heavy hitters who would no longer be able to sell health insurance products of any kind.

2. Fear of losing what you have is a great motivator in advertising, and the indemnity insurance sector of the industry exploited this sentiment to the hilt. The insurance companies hit back hard with spot advertising and targeted the government as the moral equivalent of Reagan's Evil Empire. They claimed that the Clinton plan would take away services that people already had. Warm and fuzzy images of insurance companies were presented as well as long-term and close relationships with physicians. Patients were depicted as currently having complete choice of providers. Since 85 percent of the population had coverage, this fear led to more and more people believing that the Clinton plan would hurt them. Most people agreed that health-care financing was poorly handled in the United States but also believed that they received good care. The bottom line was that the enemies of the Clinton plan depicted it as a government bureaucracy that would eliminate choice of providers.

Fearmongers used the emphasis on the employer mandate as an extension of government to pull support away from the proposed Health Security Act. The National Federation of Independent Businesses was a major organizer of manufactured grass-roots campaigns against the Health Security Act. This employer-based interest group formed an alliance with conservative voluntary associations and even talk-show hosts to exploit fear of change. (They called themselves the "No Name Coalition.") Hundreds of millions were spent in 1993 and 1994 on advertisements (especially the Harry and Louise ads), designed to build a negative constituency against reform, and in donations from political action committees (PACs) to incumbent legislators (Johnson and Broder, 1996: 53). The campaign expenditures were as large as those typically spent by a presidential candidate seeking election.

3. The later versions of reform evolved in the direction of financing through what became called the employer mandate and employer responsibility. Many of the corporate CEOs who supported health-care reform in the previous decade backed away from the Clinton plan because they did not want a fixed mandate to provide a health-care plan for their employees. Employees found fringe benefits very popular because they were untaxed sources of income, but employers always bestowed these on a voluntary basis and employees typically achieved them in collective bargaining agreements with management. The fear of mandates was based on American capital's unwillingness to be saddled with a social responsibility in an age of downsizing to face worldwide competition. Moreover, once the government established this responsibility, what would come next? The fear of precedents kept the large corporations away from the table.

Moreover, they saw the purchasing alliances, a mechanism to aggregate bargaining power or purchasers of group coverage, as a threat to their autonomy. In the past decade, many employers had lowered their health-care costs by contracting with managed care organizations. Besides, they felt they already had managed care through their health plans and so would not need to accept any proposal that smacked of regulation.

4. When bargaining time arrived, all of the major stakeholders kept holding back. The negotiation process did not take place because no stakeholders were willing to make compromises. Each remained convinced it would gain the most by being counted among the last holdouts for endorsement of the Clinton plan. The American Medical Association never got behind the plan because it was concerned about what it perceived as the Clinton plan's trend toward managed care. The American Association of Retired Persons, the biggest voluntary association in the nation, also was unenthusiastic about managed competition, fearing that its Medicare-eligible constituency would be herded into large HMOs.

5. The public rejected a potential increase in taxes to pay for the uninsured, and Congress did not want to raise taxes on the already

beleaguered middle class. The public was already paying for the care of the uninsured through high prices at hospitals and high insurance premiums, which were used for cross-subsidization. The uninsured are paid for everyday through cost-shifting. Without it, the major hospitals of this country would have to close their doors or exclude the medically indigent, a policy they could not implement legally as long as they received any federal monies for graduate medical education. Neither the public nor most employers realized that they were already paying for care for the uninsured through cost-shifting, particularly with regard to hospital *per diem* costs. Indeed, various states had created all-payer programs to make sure that hospitals gave uncompensated care and still paid their bills. The absence of the Employee Retirement Income Security Act (ERISA)-based self-insured companies from involvement at the state level in these plans meant that increasing emphasis would be placed on indemnity insurance plans to maintain their payments in these all-payer plans. The more companies went the route of self-insurance, the more likely insurance premiums would rise for group plans and individuals.

The death of health-care reform in September 1994 cleared the way for even more employers turning to managed care plans and HMOs. Employees' options shrank unless they worked in the public sector. After 1994, the number of uninsured jumped from 37 to 41 million. The states sought benefit waivers from the Health Care Financing Administration so that they could convert to capitated managed care and, in some instances, extend Medicaid benefits to a greater proportion of the population living in poverty. Market forces were turned loose, and physicians were now anxious to sign on with many managed care plans or join HMOs in order to maintain their incomes. Consumers in the millions joined the very HMOs which in 1993–1994 they claimed would keep them from maintaining relationships with their family physicians. By 1995, there were 60 million members of HMOs. And the American Association of Health Plans, the HMO trade association, estimated that by the end of 1996 there would be 70 million members. This growth is astounding because HMOs had less than 26 million enrollees in 1986.

Dramatically, in a watershed development, many of the bellwether nonprofit institutions that provided inexpensive hospital and major medical insurance in almost every state—Blue Cross and Blue Shield—now turned themselves into for-profit HMOs. In this way, they sought to compete with the new boys on the block and shed the money-losing coverage for people with preexisting serious chronic conditions whom they were forced to accept in exchange for frequent state-approved rate increases. In California, New York, and Ohio, the story was the same as the leaders of the Blues called it quits as the insurers of last resort.

The reelection of President Clinton with almost 50 percent of the vote meant an orderly transition to HMOs for the elderly and an opportunity to put forth some incremental options for expanding health insurance coverage through Medicaid and perhaps Medicare. Retiring president of the influential Commonwealth Fund, Karen Davis (1996: 831), wrote during the election campaign that

> In the absence of attention to the aggregate problem of the uninsured, special focus on vulnerable subpopulations—children, low-income women, the unemployed, and older uninsured adults—should receive greatest priority. Incremental changes that would expand health insurance coverage to groups most likely to benefit from access to care would reduce the immediate burdens created by shrinking availability of free care.

Much of her proposal would involve moderate federal expenditures that the deficit hawks in Congress would likely reject unless they heard from their constituents early and often about these modest extensions of coverage. Since Medicaid is paid for out of general revenues, an expansion of payments to the states from this source would probably have to be offset by equivalent savings. Davis does not suggest ways to create savings.

It also should be noted that Medicaid is a bargain in its coverage for healthy children. The annual average Medicaid cost in 1993 for Aid For Dependent Children was only $1057, with most of these children receiving services in fee-for-service settings. Managed care could produce an even lower average annual cost.

In fact, following the 1996 election, administration officials were considering two incremental proposals for covering uninsured children. With recent studies showing an increase in the number of uninsured children from 1987 to 1995, some thought was expressed in November 1996 about enrolling the 3 million uninsured youngsters who qualify for Medicaid but are not yet beneficiaries. In addition, to provide coverage for those youngsters who do not qualify for Medicaid but are from low-income families, a proposal was being considered to help those parents purchase private insurance (Pear, 1996: A1, A12).

At this writing, these initiatives are considered revenue-neutral because of the huge decline in the rate of increase of Medicaid expenditures in fiscal year 1995, compared to the previous five years. Some observers speculated that this reduction was due to the introduction of managed care for Medicaid beneficiaries.

While no universal coverage initiatives will be seriously proposed in Congress before the end of the millennium, the growth of managed care in Medicaid and especially in employer–employee financed health plans has put Congress in the position of regulating the relationships between health plans, their enrollees, and their physicians. Some of these concerns parallel what has already taken place in state legislatures (see Chapter 8). As James Klein, president of the Association of Private Pension and Welfare Plans (an organization that is the creation of many Fortune 500 companies), noted in late 1996: " 'Congress is going to continue its march toward becoming the nation's benefits manager, following the precedent of the mandates it imposed this year. Congress has rejected idea that employers must provide health insurance to employees. But if employers do provide coverage, Congress will specify how it should be designed' " (Pear, 1996: A12).

The national transition from fee-for-service medicine to prepaid or capitation has revealed the public's vulnerability in the health-care marketplace—even when they have access to a health plan. Managed care is an opportunity to deliver lower-cost care and brings with it the danger that complex medical care will not retain the quality achieved when cost was less of an issue.

The remainder of this work deals with how this distinctly American product—managed care—got its start, how it works, and what in the future needs to be fixed. This new and complex system of health delivery integrates what once were distinct realms, run by professional or managerial chieftains like independent fiefdoms. This very cohesiveness makes services better for the consumer and deprives the consumer of some control. It has made many of us cry, once again, in the language of our best tabloids, "There oughta to be a law against that!"

## REFERENCES

Davis, K. 1996. "Incremental coverage of the uninsured." *Journal of the American Medical Association* 276 (September 11): 831–832.

Grandy, F. 1995. "Comments on interest groups in the health care debate." Pp. 135–140 in H. J. Aaron, ed., *The Problem that Won't Go Away: Reforming U.S. Health Care Financing*. Washington, D.C.: The Brookings Institution.

Johnson, H., and Broder, D. S. 1996. *The System: The American Way of Politics at the Breaking Point*. Boston: Little, Brown.

Pear, R. 1996. "Clinton now looking at incremental approach to health-care reform." *New York Times* (November 11): A1, A12.

Wines, M., and Pear, R. 1996. "President finds benefits in defeat on health care." *New York Times* (July 30): B8.

Woodward, R. 1994. *The Agenda: Inside the Clinton White House*. New York: Simon and Schuster.

# 1
## What Is Managed Care?

Ironically, the relatively unregulated, business-dominated market that
has taken control of health care since the defeat of the Clinton plan is
proving to be a far greater threat to the autonomy of the medical profession than the elaborate apparatus of the plan could ever have been.
—Arnold S. Relman, M.D.,
former editor, *New England Journal of Medicine*
(Relman, 1996)

Managed care defies our common-sense understanding of value in the
world of work and in the area of health care. Advocates of managed
care challenge conventional wisdom when they claim that doing less
produces a greater outcome for the patient than taking action as well
as promoting the common good. Economists in the nineteenth century
believed that all work can produce something of value. Usually, the
more we do, the better off we are. Thus, more value is added to what
is produced. So when you extract iron ore from the ground and add
carbon to it under intense heat, steel is produced. For some economists,
human labor is what creates the value in the product and not just the
fact that now it can be sold in the marketplace. A similar process takes
place in protecting human life and fighting disease through medical
interventions.

In health care, if you immunize a child, that child is protected from
a disease, and the value is realized by the intervention. This is a decisive form of medical technology, which is sometimes referred to as a
preventive intervention. Managed care is a unique form of health-care
delivery because it is premised on the idea that often, in medical care,

less is more. What produces value in managed care is a good health outcome rather than medical intervention. Not every visit to a doctor is necessary; nor is every test conducted, every medication prescribed, or every placement in an intensive care unit going to produce an effective outcome. Ideally, medicine should be ruled by rationality and efficiency in the choice and implementation of evaluations and treatments. This means that the variability between providers not only should be but can be eliminated, and the only factors that should make a difference in deciding who to treat and what treatment to undertake is the nature of the patient's disease or injury.

Behind this kind of thinking is a very powerful guideline: we as a country or a planet cannot treat everything, and we need to make distinctions between treatments on the basis of effectiveness and cost. Managed care introduces explicit rationing, based on looking at an array of variables that can influence outcomes. Some treatments may be ruled out because of the patient's age or frail condition. Few surgeons would repair a hernia in a 99-year-old man. In some countries, for example, in the United Kingdom, where an effort is made to limit the amount of resources given over to health care, this kind of rationing is formulated into rules that all providers, and patients as well, must live under. Usually, these restrictions are based on scientific evidence of the limited benefit of expensive treatments for certain sectors of the population. The rules may prevent older people from gaining access to the government-run dialysis units to treat end-state renal disease. If they want to pay out-of-pocket and can afford it, they may find a private facility that can accommodate individuals with poor kidney functioning.

The complex and expensive American health-care system—with 15 percent of the population uninsured—also rations, but it is on a covert rather than an overt basis. Those without insurance use services at lower rates than those covered by any kind of health plan. But it does not follow that the young and the healthy are the uninsured. What they tend to share in common is an incapacity to afford insurance.

People without insurance are comprised of both healthy individuals and a substantial number of at-risk individuals who are underutilizers of regular sources of care. In turn, they may forego a visit to a doctor for some preventive intervention to avoid spending out-of-pocket. While not every woman who avoids a Pap smear is subject to vaginal cancer, early detection among the few who test positively for that disease saves lives as well as avoids the more costly treatments needed in advanced stages of the disease.

One also has to look at the demographics to understand why we as a nation need to cover everyone in the population. Americans constitute an aging population, and so are more subject to chronic conditions such as heart disease and cancer. An analysis of 1987 and 1990 national data found that over 45 percent of noninstitutionalized Americans have one or more chronic conditions. In the aggregate, the treatment of chronic diseases accounts for three-fourths of total health expenditures in the United States (Hoffman, Rice, and Sung, 1996). The majority of people with chronic conditions hold jobs and are not elderly. Little is known about how well managed care and health maintenance organizations provide care, not cures, for these disproportionate users of health care.

As far back as 1993, policy analysts Mark Schlesinger and David Mechanic expressed some skepticism about how well, under conditions of competition and fixed budgets, health maintenance organizations will provide for people with serious chronic illnesses and disabilities. Moreover, the potential problems identified in managed care for insuring people with chronic illnesses led these policy analysts to suggest the development of reinsurance to protect health plans; a broader benefits package than most plans offer; and sophisticated case management models (Schlesinger and Mechanic, 1993: 136).

## HEALTH MAINTENANCE ORGANIZATIONS

It has often been observed that the real consumers of health-care services are physicians rather than patients. When doctors order up tests or hospitalize patients, they encounter no financial risk in traditional fee-for-service medicine; and third-party payment softens the economic blow to the patient who might question the absolute necessity of a procedure or a hospital stay. Under third-party payment, patients freely choose providers, and there is no advance agreement to serve a particular panel of patients. Integrating payment and provider in the same plan is a key innovation in American health care because it makes discipline over physicians possible.

A health maintenance organization is both a financial plan and an organization of services for a specific population of subscribers. In this arrangement, a fiscal agent agrees to be accountable for all stipulated health services for the subscribers at a fixed price. This combination payer and provider assumes financial risk for those covered by the plan. Unlike straight indemnity insurance, HMOs exercise various kinds of control over providers and members. Those who enroll in the plan do so voluntarily and pay this price regardless of whether or not they use the services available. An advantage for the covered is that they have no first dollar or deductible obligations and generally pay only a modest co-payment when they see a doctor. In some HMO arrangements, providers do not even collect the small co-payment because it generates so little in the way of revenue and incurs an overhead cost to handle. A major component of the economic arrangements of HMOs is that all major hospital costs are paid for out of the combined capitation fees. Hospitals agree to make beds available in advance to the HMO at a discounted price or the HMO owns hospitals. Either way, HMOs try to limit hospital utilization because it is a major proportion of costs that will be taken from income.

HMOs contract with providers in various ways to get them to deliver services. In staffed HMOs, such as Kaiser-Permanente and Puget Sound, the physicians and other providers are salaried and work directly for the HMO, which also provides all nonmedical services. Doctors assume no financial risk in this model. Other arrangements use various financial incentives for either groups of physicians or solo practitioners to keep costs down.

> The group-model HMO usually provides the hospitals and other physical facilities and employs the nonphysician clinical staff. It also provides the administrative support staff. The HMO contracts with one large (professionally autonomous) multiple-specialty medical group practice for physician services. The HMO pays the medical group a monthly amount per member to provide services. (Freeborn and Pope, 1994: 21)

Within each group, usually physicians work only for that HMO, are salaried but with monetary incentives and penalties, and are at some financial risk. These groups are generally made up of a large number of physicians and provide a comprehensive set of medical services.

An expansion of the group model is called the network model, wherein an HMO contracts with several physician groups, but with the same capitation arrangements to cover members. Nonphysician services are provided by the group, which also assumes financial risk.

Finally, the fastest growing model in the 1990s is one in which individual physicians, forming an independent practice association (IPA), contract to care for covered individuals, usually on a heavily discounted fee-for-service basis. There is use of risk-capitation in some IPAs. In this model the physician often belongs to several HMOs at the same time. Located throughout a region, IPAs permit consumers to make choices from a larger number of primary-care providers and specialists than are generally found in the other models. In addition, providers are not subject to an integrated health-services system. Enrollment growth in 1994–1995 showed a 22 percent increase in networks and IPA model HMOs, compared with an 8 percent increase in staff and group model HMOs (American Association of Health Plans, 1996: 2).

HMOs are said to have a competitive advantage over traditional fee-for-service and third-party coverage because the enrolled achieve financial security as far as their medical expenses are concerned. In addition, capitation charges are considered to be lower than straight indemnification insurance policies, whether group or individual, because the provider has no incentive to do unnecessary work. Primary-care doctors or physician extenders (nurse practitioners or physician assistants) act as "gatekeepers" to specialty care. Physician extenders are much less expensive to employ than doctors and do excellent work in primary care, particularly in performing the routine but highly important tasks necessary to keep people well. A United States Office of Technology Assessment (1986) review of all studies comparing the work of nurse practitioners with physicians confirms this view.

Doctors who tend patients in managed care are driven by the concern to avoid unnecessary resource utilization. HMOs encourage patients to have regular examinations while not overusing expensive kinds of interventions. Managers of HMOs try to establish primary care as the front line of service and have an incentive to get providers to do preventive interventions and early detections through simple tests (e.g., the Pap smear) in order to avoid more complex interventions and hospitalizations later on. Sometimes providers also are given financial incentives to follow this model of service rigorously.

Although HMOs have been around for 60 years in the United States, federal legislation that provided financial incentives to start up for-profit prepaid programs initiated a rapid and enormous expansion of members in the 1980s. The Tax Equity and Fiscal Responsibility Act of 1982 expanded the market by making it easier for Medicare and Medicaid beneficiaries to enroll in HMOs. Marketing was intense. I recall that in 1984 the Chicago radio air waves were full of advertisements for HMOs, aimed at the senior citizen set. Today HMOs increasingly serve a larger and larger proportion of the over-65 population, with HMOs reporting in 1996 the development of many new Medicare risk contracts or plans to do so. Similar trends for contracts were found with regard to the Medicaid-eligible population, with many new programs coming on line.

Finding resources to deliver managed care became a less serious problem for HMOs as the market favored buyers rather than sellers of health services. The oversupply of hospital beds and physicians during the 1980s and 1990s created a strong impetus for providers to sign on with profit-making and nonprofit HMOs, guaranteeing a predictable and large volume of resources. Even august institutions found HMOs attractive. In response to losing patients, teaching hospitals with affiliations with prestigious medical schools began to create joint ventures with HMOs. In the last decade, insurance companies and state-organized Blue Cross programs began to sell HMO services to subscribers. In sum, a great transformation in the organization of providers came about with these new market considerations.

HMOs were believed to be economically viable because of their success in keeping people out of hospitals. In addition, the nonprofit HMOs essentially catered to young and healthy families, who needed routine care but rarely had the need for hospitalization. Large employers led the way in encouraging their workers to join HMOs. The financial advantage to subscribers—no deductible and no serious co-payment for office visits—was a major selling point in getting conversions from traditional insurance coverage.

Growth in HMO membership has been phenomenal during this decade. Research centers and professional associations followed these trends keenly In 1989, InterStudy, a Minneapolis-based research organization, reported that HMO membership was at 32 million. The *American Medical News* (1991: 33), a publication of the American Medical Association, noted that an American Association of Health Plans study found that HMOs appear to be most successful in the nation's largest cities and those where they have been available the longest. The cities of San Francisco (46%) and Minneapolis–St. Paul (44%) led the way with the highest numbers of HMO members among all residents.

For employers, however, some of the HMOs' great economic appeal appears to be wearing out. Even if the enrollee gives them high marks, the corporations have found that annual increases in costs can approximate those of traditional indemnification plans or even those with managed care provisions. In some cases, businesses have dropped one or more of the several HMO plans available to their employees and dependents. However, with 545 HMOs operating nationally, as reported by the Group Health Association of America (GHAA) in 1993, there seemed to be no difficulty shopping for substitute plans. Moreover, reflecting both growth and diversity, this trade association has merged with the American Managed Care and Review Association to form the American Association of Health Plans (AAHP). By late 1996 the AAHP had more than 1000 member health plans, providing coverage for over 100 million Americans nationwide.

Where did this concept come from? Is this just another foreign import, another Volkswagen or Honda? No—HMOs are a genuinely American product. One of America's major industrial magnates, Edgar Kaiser, will probably earn a place in American social history for his contribution to the extension of affordable health care to millions on the West Coast. In fact, Kaiser himself suggested that his proudest achievement was in starting the Kaiser-Permanente Health Care Partnership (Keene, 1971).

The Partnership arose from the modest need to provide modern health care in locations where such services were minimal. The urban development and agribusinesses of southern California were dependent on getting water from remote mountain areas, far distant from the coastal locations where cities were being built. Teams of construction workers were employed in the 1930s to build reservoirs and pumping stations, and to lay pipe for the aqueducts that carry water to the coastal areas and valleys. Sidney Garfield, a young physician, had tried to establish a private practice in towns near this construction. He found plenty of demand for his services among the construction crews but no way to receive adequate compensation. As a result, Garfield developed a scheme whereby each worker would contribute a small amount every week on a contract basis, paying in advance for any medical care he provided. In exchange for these payments, he agreed to provide all medical care, no matter how often it was required. Garfield even built a small mobile field hospital that could be moved on skids to follow the crews as the project advanced (Cutting, 1971: 17–18).

In 1937, some five years after Dr. Garfield started this program, Edgar Kaiser was building the Grand Coulee Dam in the state of Washington. This massive undertaking was financed out of public monies and employed large numbers of construction workers. Kaiser asked Garfield to create a health-care program for the workers and their families. This program was jointly paid for by employee and employer contributions, and it was considered a great success.

Kaiser Industries did not specialize only in dam construction. During World War II, it built cargo and troop carriers, popularly known as liberty ships. In 1942, this massive effort employed 90,000 workers in the San Francisco Bay area. Garfield was once again called upon to create a new program. After the war, the shipyard were closed and workers were dispersed. Garfield was left with a substantial group medical practice and a few thousand patients still employed by Kaiser Industries. Rather than reduce the size of the practice, he sought to keep it going by soliciting subscribers throughout the community, depending mainly on referrals (Cutting, 1971: 19). This recruitment drive was successful enough to keep the Kaiser-Permanente program going. Still known by the name of the original employer (and the site of one of his cement factories), it had 970,000 members in several states in 1970.

A similar program, the Health Insurance Program or HIP, was created in New York City in the 1940s, primarily for municipal employees. Kaiser and HIP became the models for creating financial incentives for the health maintenance organizations found in federal legislation enacted in 1973. The formation of HMOs was supported in planning grants for medical groups and loans to cover losses during the early period when subscribers were being acquired. In addition, through this legislation companies with 25 or more employees are required to offer what is called group-practice services if they have group health insurance as a fully or partially paid fringe benefit, provided an approved HMO is available in the community where the corporation is located. This enabling legislation initially created some legal problems. Some of the problems had to do with the right of a union to bargain collectively over the fringe benefits available to members, and others with the costs involved in meeting federal guidelines for planning grants and loans. Yet from these humble beginnings and encouragement from government-employed health-policy experts, the groundwork was established for the vast changes in health-care delivery we are now experiencing.

## MANAGED CARE EXPLAINED

Because it is based on rationing of services, managed care must get providers to agree to do only what is medically necessary. This does restrict the autonomy of the professional, but it is supposed to be based on outcome studies that show the efficacy of interventions. Ideally, peer review determines what is permitted and what is not, and the decision to restrict access is not made by administrators who are untrained in medical matters. The creators of contemporary managed care plans sought to eliminate the anarchy of the medical workplace, with doctors evaluating, testing, and treating in many different ways. The goal of rationing is to eliminate ineffective procedure and unnecessary treatment from the health-care system, especially if they are very costly. According to the founders of managed care, this goal can be accomplished only through the participation of providers under the same management.

Providers are linked directly to the plans that agree to deliver all medical and health services to a subscriber. Uniformity of services is necessary in order to keep costs down, and the plan, or health maintenance organization, can deliver the services at the rate it charges its customers or subscribers. Health plans hire actuaries to figure out what it will cost to deliver services to a given population, including the sick as well as the healthy. Plans are capitalized to meet state insurance commission requirements so that rationing or the HMO's closing does not occur because the plan simply miscalculated its expenditures in covering lives. While most of the original health maintenance organizations were nonprofit, this is no longer the case. Health plans are part of the commercial free enterprise system and are also run by organizations such as Kaiser-Permanente, Puget Sound, and Blue Cross/ Blue Shield. The plan makes profits when the monetary value of the resources expended is less than the revenue taken in to cover the lives of subscribers and their dependents. In financial terms, what is expended on patient care is known as the medical-loss ratio. The value of the stock of a publicly offered HMO may plunge when the news gets out that a great deal more hospitalization of patients has occurred during the last quarter of the year than was anticipated (Freudenheim, 1996). These losses reverberated in the financial markets because of the nature of financing health care in for-profit HMOs.

Whether profit making or nonprofit, the plan is paid up front, and it must live within the budget of what it takes in when it contracts to provide all medical and health services to a subscriber and dependents. Individuals who are covered by the plan pay a capitation fee, a fixed amount that provides medical services for a given period of time, regardless of the frequency of use, rather than paying fees for each service delivered. This capitation, or prepayment, creates an incentive for the providers to be cost conscious. A change in the composition of the patients recruited to the plan, known as the "case mix," can throw off the predicted service utilization.

Plans try to enroll as many healthy patients in their plans as they can so that they can deliver services at the lowest cost possible. Patients are also recruited on the basis of a contract that stresses cost containment. Under capitation, they agree to use only the panel of doctors made available by the plan. In exchange for this agreement, they have no deductible payments before their insurance becomes activated. The co-payments they make when using the doctor are very modest—usually under $10 per visit.

Providers are paid on either a capitation basis if they are primary-care providers or sometimes on a discounted fee-for-service basis. Under capitation, patients are encouraged to go as frequently as they want, while providers attempt to discourage unnecessary visits. Plans often feature a great deal of preventive services in order to avoid more expensive treatment services. Providers who deliver primary care under capitation are encouraged to see the patients with as little frequency as possible, to limit testing, and to make as few referrals to specialists as they can since they assume some financial risk. Providers who are paid on a fee-for-service basis are giving deep discounts to the plans they belong to and often have part of their fees withheld until an audit agrees that the actual visit rate and use of tests and other resources are within expected limits.

Sometimes the rules are suspended in recognition of unusual circumstances. If physicians have a disproportionately sick panel of patients, they may not be judged in the same way as all other primary-care providers; or some formula adjusted for adverse risk may be introduced to make comparisons possible with other doctors.

When hospitalization is needed, the patients must go to the hospitals approved by the plan because it has a contract with that hospital. The contract usually calls for the hospital to give a deep discount to the plan because it guarantees the hospital that a certain number of beds will be occupied. Discounting is also required of other suppliers such as pharmaceutical houses or surgical supply companies.

The new way of delivering care, through health maintenance organizations, has turned health care into a purchasable commodity. Moreover, it is produced in a more uniform and controlled work environment where there is little room for teaching and research—two of the missions of medicine—along with patient care. Each health maintenance organization is attempting to deliver a standardized product that patients would be able to recognize in any part of the world. In turn, the increasing emphasis on rationing makes it difficult for any patient to have any control in the marketplace. Since each plan is different, consumers cannot easily make careful comparisons. Moreover, consumers do not have the expertise that benefits officers in large corporations, through training and experience, have to make comparisons as to which is the better value.

HMOs operate according to standard business practices. As is the philosophy of American manufacturing, managers exhibit autocratic behavior in the workplace, and in turn, there is a kind of anarchy in the marketplace as the plans increasingly try to outdo each other in claiming they are the best. The advertisements for HMOs are starting to look like automobile ads, and this is no accident since the marketing of these health plans has become similar to marketing any mass-produced product in the United States.

How did managed care become the *plat de jour* in American health care? The table has been set by the large multinational corporations that have become intolerant of the continued rise in the cost of health care in a system of third-party payment. Today almost 60 million are covered in HMOs, and almost every group benefit package purchased by employers and paid for jointly by employees and employers has managed care features that will reduce the use of health-care services. For example, a benefits plan that allows the person covered to go directly to a specialist for a consultation will still require prior authorization if that specialist decides it's in the patient's best interest to remove a gall bladder.

With the exception of prior authorization to do an expensive procedure, the original approach to financing health care in the United States, fee-for-service, is still reproduced in the encounter between patient and doctor outside of the HMO. Some existing plans, called preferred provider organizations, continue to use the fee-for-service system but limit the person covered to their list of providers. You can go to a specialist without seeing a generalist first and the providers on the list agree to give a deep discount to the plan. Furthermore, members pay a smaller co-payment when they use a physician who participates in the plan. At the end of 1995, the AAHP estimated that 91 million enrollees and dependents were in PPOs, an increase of 12 million from 1994.

Americans continue to be very price sensitive when using health care. What managed care in its various forms has accomplished is the introduction of new reward systems for physicians and hospitals, and consumers as well, making it possible to deliver services at lower costs. These are significantly different ways of paying the doctor than are found in the American fee-for-service system. Each method of paying for medical services offers incentives to providers and patients to do certain things and avoid other things. The fee-for-service system *without* third-party payment kept the charges down because physicians were afraid to scare away patients with high fees. Patients, in turn, were careful users of the system because their post-taxed income went to pay for services. Besides, many of the encounters with physicians before the advent of antibiotics, such as penicillin, did not produce an effective or desired outcome. The technology of medicine didn't begin to get sophisticated until the 1960s. Consequently, most encounters with providers were not very expensive.

For those who could afford them as a regular source of care, doctors were attentive, courteous, and warm. In an age when physicians depended on a limited market for their services, they had to demonstrate their devotion to the few patients they had. They wished to retain patients as much as possible, and they wanted their patients to say good things about them in their neighborhoods, churches, and clubs. By keeping their fees low, doctors sought to cast as wide a net as possible to capture paying patients. In fact, general practitioners were reluctant to part with a patient through a referral to a specialist if they felt they could continue to help. Naturally, specialists knew this and expressed a great deal of gratitude for a referral because it was so hard won.

These arrangements worked to establish medicine as the major provider of health-care services to the middle classes in the United States and to promote the development of the modern acute-care voluntary hospital as we know it today (Rosenberg, 1987). By the 1930s, this system was threatened as the middle class's purchasing power declined. During the Great Depression, patients could pay neither their hospital nor their doctor bills. First, in order to keep voluntary hospital beds filled and their doors open, group hospital insurance policies were underwritten and premiums collected from subscribers. Usually, these policies were available to a workforce that expected to be steadily employed such as school teachers. Blue Cross hospital insurance was developed by the hospital industry itself as a way to keep generating income during those gloomy days. What worked in a mutually advantageous way for provider and consumer alike during hard times was even more popular during good times when more people wished to share in what became known in our popular culture as the good life. But first they were used as a way of keeping valued workers happy. Health insurance policies were offered as an across-the-board fringe benefit during World War II when wage and price freezes, compounded by a labor shortage, made it hard to retain employees without offering some reward. Then, during the postwar 1940s and 1950s, an era of substantial increases in real earnings and high progressive taxation, unionized workers sought to gain health benefits in collective bargaining agreements, sometimes in preference to increases in wages, because they were considered to be untaxed income.

The health insurance industry was off and running now, and healthcare providers were beneficiaries. First, hospital bills were paid by insurance policies and it was not too long before major medical care was also covered by indemnification policies. Benefits permitted potential patients and their providers to interact more; some of the real financial barriers to receiving medical care had been broken.

Insurance had major consequences in changing the behavior of patients and their doctors. Known as third-party payers, private insurance coverage made it possible for patients to seek doctors with great frequency, resulting in larger patient panels and more appointments per day. In fact, under these new financial conditions, which produced more patient volume, general practitioners were less reluctant to refer to specialists. The presence of coverage enhanced doctor–patient contact. For patients, insurance protected their assets since third parties paid their medical bills and they became less price sensitive. At the other end of the relationship, doctors found that increased access generated more revenues. And because their operating costs were more or less fixed, it meant more income, both relatively and absolutely, since with each additional patient seen during the day it become an increasingly profitable consultation. Moreover, access to specialists was no longer restricted by economic considerations, and each referral was less essential to their practices, but as with general practitioners, also more economically valuable than in the past. The advent of Medicare and Medicaid merely accelerated the process of growth in the industry rather than initiating it.

The explosion in health-care inflation was exacerbated by the growth of technology generated by new markets for its use. Third-party payment made consumers less price conscious in the health-care marketplace. The development of new technology means greater profits for their manufacturers as long as their products are accepted as a standard tool in the doctor's arsenal. Precisely because physicians in fee-for-service medicine become partners in owning this technology, health-policy analysts and benefits officers became unwilling to underwrite the seemingly unlimited inflation in health-care services.

The plan is fairly simple: Manufacturers of diagnostic equipment, monitoring devices, and pharmaceuticals all need to get the *real* consumer, that is, the physician, to use their products. Getting these products accepted involves efforts of persuasion comparable to the selling to any target audience of consumers. The manufacturers do have a built-in advantage, given the nature of fee-for-service medical practice in the United States. Physicians are more highly rewarded, both materially and professionally, by performing procedures rather than engaging in educational efforts with patients. Third-party payers regard these procedures as more complex than patient education and reimburse claims more handsomely when technology is used. In addition, the more procedures performed with *physician-owned* diagnostic equipment, the more financially rewarding these procedures are.

Recent studies point to the differences in the use of diagnostic equipment according to ownership by the examining physician. Moreover, the task can usually be delegated to a technician who can gain increasing proficiency in these tasks unsupervised while the physician can be doing other things. Reporting in 1991, the Florida Health Care Cost Containment Board, a state agency, found that when doctors owned their own laboratories, almost twice as many tests were performed for each patient as other laboratories. Similar results were found in this comprehensive study of the Sunshine State where the frequency of scheduled visits to physical therapy centers was higher when these facilities were owned in joint ventures by doctors (*New York Times*, August 11, 1991: E9). According to the report, 45 percent of the state's doctors were involved in such arrangements. Over 90 percent of the diagnostic imaging centers in Florida were wholly or partly owned by doctors.

The Florida report also concluded that poor and rural residents did not have improved access to these diagnostic and clinical services resulting from their proliferation around the state. This kind of finding is not limited to areas where senior citizens abound. Around the same time, a more systematic statewide study of almost 38,000 patients at 100 hospitals, reported in the *Journal of the American Medical Association*, found that patients with the same symptoms receive more diagnostic testing when they are covered by insurance than when they are not (Wenneker 1990). Massachusetts patients with chest pains or circulatory problems who were insured were more likely to be diagnosed or treated for heart disease than those patients without insurance or those covered by Medicaid. Equipment and staff time are sometimes used selectively so that the procedures ordered up will yield revenues. Similarly, patients who are eligible for Medicaid yield lower returns for the same diagnostic procedures as those who are insured or covered by the Medicare program and, consequently, also receive less testing.

Paralleling the extension of technology as part of the relationship with patients was the development of life-extending technology for those near death. Respirators were originally designed for and used with patients who had lung surgery, allowing these organs to recover slowly. Additional uses were found in intensive care units for this equipment, and patients who were in critical condition, with multiple organ failures, were placed on respirators.

Following the scholarly exposé in a major medical journal on involuntary clinical experimentation initiated by Beecher (1966), in which he cited numerous studies where patients never gave informed consent to participate in dangerous experiments, federal legislators and patient rights advocates began to wonder about how much choice patients had in undergoing clinical procedures or treatment regimens that might be futile, invasive, or even have adverse side effects. The development of informed consent for standard clinical care followed on the heels of similar protocols to protect the rights of subjects in experiments. Not surprisingly, consumers began to wonder whether they were being told everything or whether doctors knew how to communicate with patients. However, it was undoubtedly the crisis of rising health-care costs that spurred medical ethicists to begin to see that patients had little choice to refuse these invasive procedures with questionable efficacy.

Now device manufacturers face harder times, as the HMOs take a close look at how much they need in the way of expensive technology. Where once technology was moved quickly into office and hospital-based practice, today providers and payers want to know what is necessary and what works (Borzo, 1996: 4). The reduction in fee-for-service medicine, combined with third-party payment, is finally reducing the demand for new technology.

When third-party payment augments but does not replace the classic fee-for-service relationship between doctors and patients, it still means some out-of-pocket costs for routine office visits. The concept of insurance was a way to protect against major economic catastrophes that could befall a family, such as results from the death of the major wage earner, the loss of a home, or the loss of a business. Some consumers and a few providers became concerned about the high cost of services rendered. Models for how to rein in out-of-pocket expenditures did exist, although the American Medical Association severely disapproved of doctors who worked for a salary—the keystone of the first-generation HMOs that provided comprehensive care for a single fee paid up front.

Kaiser and other early health maintenance organizations delivered good services at moderate cost to the membership. In so doing, consumers "locked in" their health-care costs for an entire year through this prepayment arrangement with specific providers. Not only were doctors services available under these plans, but also hospital care was provided for a single fee, with the provider assuming the financial risk if there was an unexpected utilization.

Ever since the 1960s, employers have been concerned about controlling their expenditures for health care and have looked for ways to avoid increases in the costs of services. In addition, consumers have tried to lock in their annual costs for health care. Today in HMO programs, a group of doctors, including specialists, provide all the medical specialties and services by contract to a number of patients who will be cared for, no matter how frequently or infrequently they use the services. In addition, hospital-based services are also part of the contracted benefits and are prearranged by contracts between HMOs and hospitals or by outright purchase or building of hospitals exclusively dedicated to care for subscribers.

Skills learned in business schools and cost-based planning drive HMOs today. Contemporary HMOs are less likely to be staffed by salaried physicians who work in HMO-owned offices and hospitals and are more likely to be part of a network of providers. The overcapacity of the hospital system has made it possible for HMOs to drive hard bargains with community hospitals and academic medical centers to admit their patients, when appropriate, at a rate well below that charged the indemnity insurance companies.

Cost-consciousness is raised to a high art in managed care organizations. Managed care will pay for low-cost preventive medicine, early detection and treatment of disease, and health promotion activities such as smoking-cessation programs. Marketing is toward those already healthy, focusing on health-promotion activities such as discounted memberships in fitness centers, rather than showing how well they care for stroke victims. It limits benefits where decision makers regard the care as pure comfort and not always medically necessary, as in the case of hospital stays for psychiatric care and unlimited psychotherapy. Care coordination for complex cases may also be part of an HMO's way of making sure that physicians do not order unnecessary care. Service substitution also takes place, as when nurse practitioners and physician assistants provide primary care under the supervision of a physician or when outpatient care is given instead of hospitalizing the patient.

In sum, managed care means that the providers are watched carefully to make sure they do not provide unnecessary care. Medical care is also rationed through prior authorization mechanisms, a form of micromanagement that professionals thoroughly resent. Even before a sick person gets to the point of needing some expensive specialty-based procedure, the primary-care provider is performing gatekeeping functions in the HMO, making sure that when a specialist is seen it is truly for something that the primary-care provider cannot do.

By stressing prevention and early intervention, HMOs are able to deliver comprehensive services at reasonable costs. Certainly, HMOs have an admirable record with regard to childhood immunizations. Yet there is another side to medical practice, and that involves care when a person is seriously ill. Critics of HMOs suggest that seeing fewer specialists is not necessarily a good thing, especially if you suffer from a serious chronic condition or disability. Moreover, in many HMOs, specialty services may be available at "centers of excellence," but they are not accessible because they are not near where subscribers live. Plan financial agents may develop contracts with facilities that provide deep discounts, but because they deal with rare diseases they may be far from a given patient's home community and therefore cannot always accommodate routine family needs, including being able to hold on to one's job. One North Carolina family underwent total disruption when a child required bone marrow transplants, which were available only under the plan in Baltimore, Maryland (Weston and Lauria, 1996). As Harry and Louise might say in their famous 1993 commercial for the status quo, "There's got to be a better way."

The market road to cutting costs in health care has done little to make the American citizen feel more secure knowing that unregulated competition was in the driver's seat. Since 1992, with this enormous growth in HMO membership and the addition of managed care features to indemnity insurance policies, the public has not regarded these changes as beneficial. A public opinion poll conducted by the *New York Times* in June 1996—three and a half years into the Clinton administration and two years after the failure of health-care reform legislation—nearly one-third of the 1121 people surveyed—32 percent—said that health care had gotten worse since Mr. Clinton became president. Only 12 percent said it had gotten better (Wines and Pear, 1996: B8). Blame for the decline in quality was laid at the doors of the big insurance companies and the big HMOs and not the president. And the public got it right when it said that the failure to enact universal health insurance was due to the stonewalling of the Republicans in 1993 and 1994 on health care and the Republican Congress elected in 1994. The small-business lobby was overjoyed that it didn't get an employer mandate to provide insurance, and the big corporations were seeing their costs hold steady, if not decline, as more and more employees chose the option of reducing their choices.

## REFERENCES

American Association of Health Plans. 1996. *1995–1996 AAHP HMO and PPO Trends Report.* http://www.aahp.org/LI/RESEARCH.

American Medical News. 1991. "HMOs successful in big cities, old markets." *American Medical News* (February 18): 33.

Beecher, H. K. 1966. "Consent in clinical experimentation: Myth and reality." *Journal of the American Medical Association* 195 (January 3): 34–35.

Borzo, G. 1996. "Managed care and technology assessment: Who should pay?" *Technology News* (March): 3–4.

Cutting, C. 1971. "Historical development and operating concepts." Pp. 17–22 in Anne R. Somers, ed., *The Kaiser-Permanente Medical Care Program.* New York: Commonwealth Fund.

Freeborn, D. K., and Pope, C. R. 1994. *Promise and Performance in Managed Care: The Prepaid Group Practice Model.* Baltimore: Johns Hopkins University Press.

Freudenheim, M. 1996. "Market place: HMOs are having trouble maintaining financial health." *New York Times* (June 19): D12.

Hoffman, C., Rice, D., and Sung, H. Y. 1996. "Persons with chronic conditions: Their prevalence and costs." *Journal of the American Medical Association* 276: 1473–1479.

Keene, C. 1971. "Kaiser Industries and Kaiser-Permanente health care partnership." Pp. 13–16 in Anne R. Somers, ed., *The Kaiser-Permanente Medical Care Program.* New York: Commonwealth Fund.

New York Times. 1991a. "When doctors own their own labs." *New York Times* (August 11): E9.

Relman, A. 1996. "What went wrong with the Clinton Health Plan." *New England Journal of Medicine* 335 (August): 601–602.

Rosenberg, Charles. 1987. *The Care of Strangers: The Rise of America's Hospital System.* New York: Basic Books.

Schlesinger, M., and Mechanic, D. 1993. "Challenges for managed competition from chronic illness." *Health Affairs* 12 (Supplement): 123–137.

U.S. Office of Technology Assessment. 1986. *Nurse Practitioners, Physician Assistants and Certified Nurse-Midwives: A Policy Analysis.* Technology Case Study 37. Washington, D.C.: U.S. Government Printing Office.

Wenneker, M. B. 1990. "The association of payer with utilization of cardiac procedures in Massachusetts." *Journal of the American Medical Association* 264, 10 (September 12): 6–11, 1255–1260.

Weston, B., and Lauria, M. 1996. "Patient advocacy in the 1990s." *New England Journal of Medicine* (February 22): 334–335.

Wines, M., and Pear, R. 1996. "President finds benefits in defeat on health care." *New York Times* (July 30): A1, B8.

# 2
# American Business Falls in Love with Managed Care

> If we are going to control costs, we need a system in which the decision makers feel pressure to provide high quality care and control costs.
> —David Eddy, Duke University
> (Freudenheim, 1992)

The dramatic shift to managed care is the equivalent of turning around an entire fleet of battleships in a narrow strait. Never before has the American health-care system undergone such fundamental financing and organizational changes in the delivery of services. One health-policy analyst, Ed O'Neil, has likened what has happened to the equivalent of the collectivization of agriculture in the Soviet Union in the 1930s. This analogy seems fitting because many of the formerly independent providers are now linked in systems that dictate how they shall be productive. It is a tremendous achievement to turn the health-care industry around in such a short period of time, although it may not be a system that is good for the chronically ill or disabled, especially if they do not live near the services they require. And it certainly is a reversal of fortune for specialists in the United States.

Managed care is driven by concern for cost and an oversupply of physicians, making it possible to persuade some, at least, to learn to work within a cost-conscious environment. In addition, an oversupply of hospital beds encouraged HMOs to contract with hospitals and thereby avoid investment in hospital construction, making it less expensive to get off and running as a service provider since there was no wait for hospitals to be built or for loans to be acquired. Moreover, in this land of corporate enterprise, no great public uproar arose over shifting health care to vertically integrated providers who sought to deliver services and make a profit on that service. The markets from managed care were there, and the profits based on efficient use of services were there to be taken. In addition, the value of the stock of the publicly traded HMOs appreciated substantially in a short period of time. Salaries and bonuses for CEOs in this industry reflected these changes in economic value. The demand for executives who can negotiate capitation or other risk-bearing payment arrangements with physician groups or networks increased enormously in the mid-1990s (Pallarito, 1995: 30).

Building on the base provided by large employers who are looking to rein in their costs, the recruitment of subscribers has not ebbed. Currently, HMOs are signing up small employers in great numbers (Salak, 1995). HMOs will be recruiting senior citizens and even creating profit-making entities to provide managed care for those eligible for Medicaid. What it won't do is provide care for the uninsured since HMOs creatively avoid giving uncompensated care. In addition, as a number of health-policy analysts have pointed out in medical journals, HMOs have not agreed to underwrite the costs of graduate medical education in the United States, an important function previously undertaken by academic medical centers creatively. They would put together public funding through Medicare and Medicaid and private surpluses from indemnity insurers to provide cross-subsidies for uncompensated care. Thus, in the 1980s and 1990s, few of the uninsured were turned away when they needed urgent care.

The story of HMOs is no longer confined to health-care journals and their policy wonks. The subject of America's best HMOs made the cover of *Newsweek* (June 24, 1996). Almost a year earlier, Ellyn Spragins in the October 1995 *Bloomberg Personal*, a *parvenu* among magazines, found HMOs reluctant to give out information on how they compensate their doctors, the rate of doctor turnover, their certification by national boards, or the amount they spend on patient care from the revenues generated by capitation payments. Note that these articles are not discussions of the country's best surgeons or best hospitals, but a rating of integrated health systems—which up to 1994 was not even conceivable.

All this is possible because the captains of corporations decided they had to say no to the steadily growing demands for services or, more significantly, our potential for outrunning the resources to pay for them. Most of this was done out of pure self-interest, not the public interest. As prices keep rising in health care, often due to the introduction of new technology, the nation's productivity cannot expand rapidly enough to absorb all these new expenses. Part of the problem relates to our success as a nation in keeping down the birth rate and slowing the death rate. Demography appears to be destiny as far as the cost of health care is concerned. The American population in general, and the workforce in particular, is aging.

The belief in unrestrained economic growth as the answer to all problems is wearing out its welcome, even in this age of resurgent capitalism. But the market is a powerful idea when viewed as the solution to the growing costs of health care in the United States. The CEOs and chairs of the boards of directors of our most prosperous corporations have decided to reject government-generated solutions as too regulatory and too likely to impose mandates on employers, even when they voluntarily share the cost of health plans with employees. The Clinton health-care reform plan seemed to open up fears of regulation in business life. This occurred even though less than 10 years ago U.S. business leaders considered a national health insurance program as a practical solution to their problems (Freudenheim, 1990). It is not that business leaders have become the new socialists in America, although some corporations—to survive—were happy in the 1970s (e.g., Chrysler) to be bailed out through government-guaranteed loans. They were facing inflation and did not feel they could control it on their own. A 1990 corporate survey found an average cost for health care of $3217 per worker, a 17.1 percent increase from 1989 (Freudenheim, 1991: D1). Even a reduction of the increase for the following year, let us say from 17 to 10 percent, would involve enormous savings. Yet the managed care solutions undertaken by individual corporations often further unraveled the health-care system as less cross-funding remained available to cover the costs of uncompensated care for the uninsured.

The gravy years for hospitals and doctors set the stage for the current corporate rebellion. Concern with runaway expenses began to be expressed 20 years ago when increasing competition from other countries made profits less predictable than in the past. Starting in the late 1970s, employers began to address the problem of health-benefit costs. A labor–management group came out with a position paper on the subject, endorsing an early version of prospective payment systems for hospitals, managed care, and outcome studies to determine the cost effectiveness of different types of treatment. When it was discovered that the productivity of American industry declined during the 1970s, the business moguls who competed with international companies that sold similar commodities sought to cut their production costs. Comparisons of Japanese and American labor costs in the automobile industry in 1983 found comparable wage rates, but the fringe benefit package made American labor costs expensive: on an hourly basis, total U.S. labor costs were 60 percent higher (Thurow, 1984: 1569). Economists pointed out almost a decade ago that Japanese plant investment, double that of American industry, helped account for greater productivity.

Modernization for the American auto industry may be held back by added financial burdens for health-care benefits. Cash reserves that could be used to secure loans may go to pay for health care for aging employees or retired workers. This cry of pain is heard around the world.

The future growth and competitiveness of our economy are also being jeopardized by these expenses as well as present capital requirements. American allocations for civilian research and development in the United States were lower than those in Japan and in other major industrial powerhouses. In the current decade, a congressional report showed it to be in further comparative decline (Broad, 1992: C1). In addition, the human capital of the American economy was seen as inferior. American workers were viewed as poorly educated compared to their counterparts in major competing nations.

The education system in the United States failed to establish uniform standards for all, and this meant that our labor force was inconsistent as far as basic literacy and mathematic skills were concerned. Leaders of business in the United States, seeking to find funds to remedy these national deficits, found health benefits a likely target. This became the cash cow they needed to become competitive, influencing all kinds of corporate thinking, sometimes with unintended negative consequences.

The health-care inflation of the 1980s impacted on corporate decisions, making it more advantageous to move away from the Northeast and Midwest. Relocated in the Sun Belt in order to lower their wage rate, real estate costs, and taxes, corporations have found that health benefits are even more expensive there than in the older industrial states of the Rust Bowl. As in other places, health-care providers seek to cross-fund their operations to make up for reduced incomes from Medicare or Medicaid patients. Companies that moved southward also found more for-profit companies running hospitals and diagnostic centers, with high fees and frequent referrals by providers. The financing system is interdependent, despite multiple funding sources. Corporations can run but cannot hide from burdensome health-benefit costs. The segmentation of the financing of care for the elderly and the poor did not prevent providers, or in some cases state plans, to seek to make up the difference from the patients with better coverage. Indeed, there was a health-care system and there was no escaping its distortions.

Trends in the annual growth in corporations' payments for health benefits as a share of pretax profits pointed to similar conclusions. Over a 22-year period, these costs increased sixfold and they also became a greater part of labor costs, increasing from 2.1 percent in 1965 to 6.2 percent in 1987. Despite the opportunity to deduct these costs from corporate taxes, the managers of large businesses must factor them into the price of cars or any other product, when offering them for sale. Consequently, it is increasingly more difficult to compete in the world market with other corporations that do not have to bear these expenses.

Escape from the interdependence of the financing system is remote for all the players in this game. The workforce also bears an increasing burden for the cost of Medicare, an item deducted from the paychecks of the currently employed to pay for the care of the population over 65 years of age, and for some younger beneficiaries in special categories, for example, people in need of dialysis because of kidney failure. The funds necessary to pay for people eligible for Medicare increases substantially every year. Readers with a Social Security account need only examine the last 10 years: when disaggregated from the Social Security pension section, the amount that goes for Medicare increases a great deal annually, even when annual income does not increase at the same rate. In addition, employers contribute to Medicare up through the same amount of covered wages. This is an additional contribution for employers from their cash reserves.

What becomes clearly irrational, and a growth-retarding factor, is how the country's health-care financing system becomes a restraint on occupational and geographic mobility for those seeking advancement and change of employment. The high cost of health-care services has made members of the workforce reluctant to leave jobs with good benefit packages. As the cost of care increases, workers look to protect and hold on to their existing benefits, creating what is popularly known as "job lock." A 1991 New York Times/CBS News Poll found that "three in ten Americans say they or someone in their household have at some time stayed in a job to keep the health benefits" (Eckholm, 1991: A1). Passed in 1996, the bipartisan Kassebaum–Kennedy bill should reduce some of the American workers' reluctance to take new jobs since under this new law their benefits will now be more portable.

Loss of employment also creates barriers to care for workers who can least afford it. Job turnover becomes a health and financial problem when workers lose employment. Some Americans change jobs with great frequency, particularly in agriculture, construction, repair, entertainment, and personal services. The current dependence on employment-based health benefits becomes unworkable from the point of view of maintaining the health of members of the workforce and their dependents. Even when federal law mandates that former employees be allowed to retain coverage by direct payment of premiums, sometimes these expenses are beyond the means of many families. Can a family of two or three with an income of $20,000 per year pay directly for health insurance and also cover other necessities such as housing and food (Schorr, 1990)?

## INTRODUCING LIMITS

As health insurance became less affordable to the near-poverty population, several states attempted to address this problem. But the prime aim of corporations, insurance companies, and the managers of the Medicare and Medicaid system as well is to restrain utilization. Health-care services experts in the United States agree that there was unlimited demand for services when third-party coverage was in place. As everyone knows, making more use of something good will drive up the cost. In the case of health care, insurance premiums increase when we all use services covered by those policies. But self-restraint is difficult to manage when we know the services we seek are going to be paid for. The logic was that if something was paid for, it would be provided, even when it was marginally useful to the patient. Patients and providers were seen as being in collusion, giving the ultimate payers—employers, Social Security payers, or general taxpayers—no hope in containing costs.

Lester Thurow (1984: 1570) captures the self-perpetuating and expansive nature of such an interlocked system of incentives to spend and use, use and spend.

> In these circumstances an insurance system ends up having no constraints. Insurance companies have an interest in higher health-care expenditures, since higher expenditures lead to higher corporate incomes. Doctors practicing in a fee-for-service system have a personal interest in prescribing services, since they raise their own income by doing so, and in an insurance system doctors know that they will not be directly raising costs for their patients if they do so. With insurance, patients have no interest in restraining their own health-care expenditures. The result, not surprisingly, is a system with exploding expenditures.

Efforts by employers to save money on health benefits have created a different way of defining benefits. In fact, employers seek to define not benefits but costs. In so doing, they are looking to gain assistance from employees.

## COST-SHIFTING AND OTHER MOVES BY EMPLOYERS

Employers first looked for relief in the way the health-benefit package was paid for. Employers therefore started to introduce or significantly increase payments for health benefits taken from employees' earnings on a paycheck-by-paycheck basis. By 1990, 82 percent of companies surveyed required that workers pay part of their family health-care costs. Business writer Milton Freudenheim (1990: D9) reported that "individual employees contributed $396 a year on average, up 43.5 percent, from $276 in 1989, while family payments rose 29 percent to $1,068." There was considerable variation in costs within different types of businesses. Industries (e.g., utilities) with older and unionized workers had higher costs than those with younger nonunionized employees (e.g., retail and wholesale).

Employer-based health insurance was always a better deal than purchasing insurance individually. The premiums for group policies were lower than those for individual policies because of two factors. First, it is cost effective for insurance underwriters to prepare and market a policy for a group than for an individual; and second, the underwriters use experience-rating rather than community-rating data on risks to determine the price of the insurance to the buyer of group insurance, usually producing considerable savings. Policies that were originally written to cover all expenses for beneficiaries rapidly went out of style.

Next, benefits officers followed the example of Medicare in making beneficiaries more accountable for their own behavior in using health-care services unnecessarily. Employers began to get insurance underwriters to include deductible and co-payment requirements for all those covered. In a process designated cost-shifting, beneficiaries were now required to pay the first dollar amounts on all health care during a 12-month period before the benefits were activated. These provisions usually involved $100 or $200 per person or no more than $400 annually per family. Co-payment meant that any visit to the doctor involved some sharing of the cost by the patient, which was usually set at 20 percent of the doctor's fee. The policy underwriters recognized that rare but unexpected financial responsibilities for the covered individual or family could become burdensome. Most policies stated that after those covered by the benefits accumulated substantial out-of-pocket payments, the insurance usually covered all other charges at 100 percent. Benefits were also limited by an upper cap on how many dollars would be paid out over a lifetime or annually for beneficiaries.

To what extent would such changes in cost-shifting endanger the health of people who did not previously face any financial barrier to services? Did those who had complete coverage for all services and had no financial responsibility overuse services? The answers to these questions were provided by an elaborate experimental study involving thousands of families who were randomly assigned to different types of insurance coverage, ranging from some types with no cost or minimal costs to the subjects in the study to others with substantial financial deductibles and co-payment requirements.

The Rand Health Insurance Experiment analyzed data for 3539 persons aged 17 to 61 in order to determine the effect of cost-sharing on seeking care for serious and minor symptoms. Annually, the managers of this study administered a survey in which they asked whether the randomly assigned participants to different types of coverage had serious and minor symptoms during the past month and whether they saw a physician. Physician panelists judged whether symptoms were of either category, with the understanding that a serious symptom (e.g., chest pains while exercising) warranted care while a minor system (e.g., stomach flu or virus with nausea or vomiting) was deemed as not severe or not necessary to bring to the attention of a doctor or other primary-care provider. The summary of the findings is most interesting for understanding the direction businesses have gone in restricting benefits for their employees:

> The cost-sharing group was nearly one third less likely than the free-care group to see a physician when they had minor symptoms. The free-care and cost-sharing groups do not differ significantly in seeking care for serious symptoms. (Shapiro, Ware, and Sherbourne, 1986: 246)

Confirmation of these results came from another study of HMO utilization, wherein it was found that a modest co-payment of $5 per visit reduced use of primary-care services by 11 percent at the Group Health Cooperative of Puget Sound, a Seattle HMO (Cherkin, 1989).

The most vulnerable participants, the chronically ill and the poor, responded to these incentives or disincentives to use services much in the same way as those who were better off or had no serious chronic conditions. Interestingly, participants with low income and serious chronic illnesses responded differently in terms of frequency of serious symptoms. The free-care group reported a reduction of symptoms from the time of the inception of the study, whereas the cost-sharing group showed an actual increase. In this study and others, poorer persons with hypertension had adverse effects from participation in cost-sharing insurance schemes.

Employers searched for other ways of saving money besides passing on costs to their employees. All these measures involved asserting greater control over what services would be paid for. Large companies also found it possible to assert direct control over the health-benefit program itself to limit costs, eliminating the need for insurance companies. Some changes in federal law provided the enabling legislation for these measures.

## SELF-INSURING UNDER ERISA

Some large companies took advantage of the provisions of the 1974 Employee Retirement Income Security Act (ERISA) to emancipate themselves from the rules of state insurance commissions that set up mandated benefits in health-care policies and from the costs of purchasing insurance in the marketplace. While most of the mandated benefits should be applauded (e.g., coverage of pregnancy), some might be considered frills (e.g., acupuncture). ERISA also made it possible for the self-insured to avoid taxes on premiums. The self-insurance statutes meant that large corporations with sufficient cash reserves or borrowing power could essentially pay for the benefits of their employees without a policy. They usually did this by establishing a trust fund dedicated to paying for claims made under their health-benefit plans. Because ERISA preempts state legislation, states currently do not regulate the 36 percent of the insurance business that stems from the directly self-insured and reinsurance for the self-insured. Reinsurance means that the self-insured purchase policies to stop losses in the case of catastrophic illnesses requiring extraordinary payments to providers. The employee claims still need to be processed, and corporations contract for these services from insurance companies with trained and available personnel to do this task. In sum, what the large corporations saved was the cost of underwriting and the profits that would go to the insurers.

Part of the premium for insurance in the United States goes to pay for uncompensated care given by hospitals. In some states, hospitals have been bailed out this way because in the absence of these institutions, paying or insured patients would have no place to go. Without these plans to take from the rich to pay for the poor, hospitals that give charity care or do not collect fully from patients without insurance will run up such burdensome debts that they will be in danger of closing their doors. These state-based plans are called all-payer mechanisms to keep providers of free care solvent. Critics of ERISA argue that companies which operate their health-benefit programs under this federal statute are not making contributions to maintaining the providers who give uncompensated care or basic health insurance for those with serious chronic illnesses. The self-insured do not help subsidize the uninsured by supporting the all-payer programs. Nor do they contribute to the state-based high-risk pools to make insurance available at moderate costs to those with preexisting conditions.

Self-insuring has not produced enormous savings for the companies that have gone that route. However, since these companies usually have an older workforce than that found among all employers, their expenditures perhaps would be even higher without self-insurance. In general, these firms have not cut back on important benefits, despite their freedom from state insurance laws.

Approximately 46 percent of all the employer-based health-benefit plans in the United States are self-insured, according to the U.S. Department of Labor. Typically, self-insured plans are similar to purchased group insurance, having basic and major medical coverage, combining them in a single set of comprehensive benefits.

## PREFERRED PROVIDER NETWORKS

A concept gradually emerged among businesses and insurance carriers wherein employees were marketed and sold to the lowest-bidding providers. The power of guaranteeing large numbers of users has been persuasive to doctors and hospitals worried about maintaining their market shares. A preferred provider organization (PPO) is a way of developing a network of hospitals, physicians, and other health services who are willing to give a discount to the payer on the fees charged for services. To get employees to prefer these providers to any provider they choose, the plans that build in a PPO feature usually reduce the user's deductibles and co-payments. Sometimes the employee contribution to premiums is also reduced to create an incentive to use the network's providers. Insurers or the plan managers for self-insured corporations negotiate to get providers to agree to participate at the discounted rates, usually with the anticipation that they will increase their patient volume.

Under the PPO plan, employees still go to any provider they wish outside of the network, although they pay more for those services. Thus, freedom of choice is still maintained. But in some plans there may be a network without much networking. Although price reduction is achieved, few networks work in a coordinated fashion to reduce utilization, as in the case of HMOs or IPAs with primary-care providers acting as "gatekeepers" to the specialty services.

Participating companies in PPO arrangements were watched very closely in the 1980s and 1990s because they were viewed as the wave of the future. The Pepsico Corporation, Southwestern Bell, and American Telephone and Telegraph are among those companies that have gone the route of establishing provider networks that can save employees money if they are used. These companies reckoned that the increases in their health-care bill were 20 percent less than if they had not made the PPO available to workers (Kramon, 1989b: D2).

Feedback from employees and their families is also a way of evaluating the PPO. Southwestern Bell surveyed its employees and families to determine whether there was consumer satisfaction with the PPO: 82 percent of the 6800 people who used the network thought the care was very good, and 36 percent thought the care was better than in the past. Not everyone, however, who tried this scheme was happy with it. Some older people with serious chronic illnesses were dissatisfied with the plan itself because doctors whom they wished to retain were not part of the network. Those employees or family members paid more for services and also cost the company more because they exercised freedom of choice.

There may be a lesson here for future network constructors. It should be noted that since older workers are the most frequent users of expensive services (e.g., open-heart surgery), it would be most effective in accomplishing the goal of cost control for health benefits if they could have their doctors in the network. Perhaps the way to plan a PPO is to start with a profile of the employees and families who cost the most in claims and sign on their doctors.

Despite high levels of consumer satisfaction experienced by the basically healthy people who use PPOs, these plans still create some confusion because there are doctors who leave PPOs and in some areas participants in the network are few and far between. Nevertheless, the holder of the purse strings who can guarantee access to a large number of patients is generally able to set prices in today's medical markets. It has been observed that

> the ability of large purchasers to gain increased control over the conditions of their purchase of medical care comes in part from the fact that the element in shortest supply in the health care system is no longer hospital beds or physicians but patients who have the means to pay for care—insured patients. (Gray, 1991: 258)

This same search for savings has led to the modification of PPOs, so that users of the network now have to go through a primary-care provider who acts as a gatekeeper to specialty care. In addition, utilization review, including preadmission review, has also been added to the benefit requirements in most PPOs. This may sound very familiar to readers, as different types of programs designed to save money are grafted on to each other. The use of managed care provisions makes the PPO similar to those HMOs defined in Chapter 1 as independent practice associations.

An interesting joint venture of almost quasi-experimental proportions took place in 1988 between an insurance company that put together a nationwide PPO for an electronics equipment manufacturer. The Cigna Corporation underwrote a policy for health benefits for Allied-Signal, a corporation with 76,000 employees, to guarantee that costs for employees enrolled in their PPO network would not increase by more than 10 percent a year. The PPO arrangements included case management features. Cigna also made similar guarantees on increases in costs for the employees who were outside of the network— that is, that costs would not increase more than 15 percent a year. Cigna and Allied-Signal were thrilled when increases for the PPO came in well under their estimates. However, guarantees on costs for the Allied-Signal workforce *not* in the PPO was a losing proposition for Cigna (Kramon, 1989a: D2). Do providers compensate for loss of volume to PPOs or reductions in price when they do join networks by making it up on those traditionally insured?

Limiting choice but producing savings to the consumer is the theme of other efforts to cut health-benefit expenditures for the corporation in America. A joint venture in savings then is also the rationale of employers offering an HMO option to employees in their "menu" of health benefits. The mutual interest of employers and employees in cutting utilization has led to the impressive growth of HMOs in their various forms. Now small companies are offering a managed care option and sometimes as the only plan they will provide employees (Salak, 1995: 31).

There is some evidence that the savings realized on HMOs is only temporary. Health reporter Sue Shellenbarger (1990: B4) offered the following explanation as to why the cost of HMOs seems to be chasing the cost of traditional health insurance plans. First, until recently federal rules required that employers make equal contributions to the HMO and non-HMO plans, thus encouraging HMOs to base their rates on what was charged by indemnity plans and not on their costs. Second, and most important, the HMO movement introduced a boosting effect on the rates for conventional insurance coverage. According to Shellenbarger,

> HMOs attract younger employees, according to most employers, leaving older workers in conventional insurance plans. That means that premiums for conventional plans rose even faster than they would have without HMOs—dragging up HMO and total costs with them. (B4)

This kind of "creaming off" of the healthy (and the young) is a similar process as that identified in the way PPOs may save money for employers or insurers for some of the workforce covered but not for others in conventional plans where charges are driven up.

## BUSINESS SEEKS TO UNIFY

Experts on controlling expenditures on health-care benefits agree that several things can be done to rein in costs. Payers can attempt to negotiate over price, as in the case of seeking to develop networks of providers who offer services at a discount. An oversupply of providers and facilities produces a market in which the buyer has great advantages. You can restrict access to certain services to specific locations where it is cheaper to deliver them, such as tests, diagnostic procedures, or minor surgeries. Providers willing to break away from standard practices will be more than willing to do this, particularly if they are competing for market share with other providers and they can deliver at a lower price by doing things through ambulatory care. Prior authorization is also a way to avoid expensive claims where the service proposed is not necessary or appropriate. Again, provider surplus makes for compliance in managed care arrangements. Managed care increases administrative expenses for providers, a cost that is passed on to payers. Finally, it is possible to limit payment for "big-ticket" items that are sometimes not successful or may need to be redone. Heart, liver, and kidney transplants are not always indicated but are always very expensive. A year's worth of all medical care and drugs before, during, and after a heart transplant averages over $160,000.

Employers are learning to say no and are also learning that they can do more together than separately. The concern over the introduction of Relative Value Scales (RVS), the new way of paying doctors under Medicare, is representative of how they cannot overcome their problems individually. Benefits officers are worried that providers will increase their fees to compensate for losses in income engendered by this system of payment for Medicare patients, which rewards physicians for consultation and educational activities with patients more and reduces payments for doing technical procedures and surgery. There is fallout for all payers because of the unintended interdependence in the system brought about by providers taking protective action in the face of regulatory changes. Eventually, the private payers will jump on the bandwagon and use this new fee schedule, as they did with the introduction of Diagnostic Related Groups or DRGs. However, the short-term results will likely create even greater burdens for those considered to have the ability to pay.

By 1985 the ideology of free enterprise and avoidance of government interference with business gave way to pragmatic concerns about competitiveness in the global economy. Corporate America appeared close to be willing to sacrifice the private health insurance industry, and the free enterprise that it represents, for relief from the increasing burden of health-benefit costs. Facts are stubborn things, and the business leaders were starting to shed their ideological blinders in search of survival, if not excellence. Like former Soviet leaders who are now proto-capitalists, some members of the world of free enterprise are looking for collective solutions.

Today the stress for big business produced by our health-care system is exacerbated by old commitments to retired employees. These obligations have now been declared debts. Recent changes in accounting rules require new ways of identifying future medical benefits to retired workers. In 1993 corporations began to charge the medical obligations of future retirees as a debit against income. This change impacts on the profit statements of corporations, which is not just a change on paper but can affect the way investors approach the purchase of stocks and bonds that are issued. Some corporations are preparing to meet retirees' needs by setting up trust funds, with others taking a wait and see attitude concerning the overall financing of the American health-care system. The possibility of lost benefits for retired workers, or drastically reduced packages, has pushed some employers, and especially unions under the banner of the AFL-CIO to energetically seek the creation of national health insurance.

A good number of American business leaders are beginning to see that the segmented payment and delivery system is working against them, since controls introduced in Medicare and Medicaid mean increases in prices for services for those covered by private insurance. Cost-shifting is not solely something that employers do with employees. It is also the case that when certain procedures are restricted to an outpatient setting, the cost of maintaining inpatient settings increases to make up for the loss of volume. It has gotten to the point that payers have taken note of the enormous cost involved in supporting a premature infant in an intensive care unit and have begun to realize that paying for prenatal care is a very cost-effective idea. Insurance was always organized to deal with low risks but very expensive losses. Now benefits officers are redefining how to deal with preventable losses up front rather than paying for expensive hospital stays and procedures later on.

Pure self-interest is driving our business class into the arms of the HMOs, but they may not be able to escape blame for what might occur in the future. A government-financed health-care system once appealed to corporations because they viewed rationing decisions of expensive procedures to be on the horizon and they did not wish to be responsible for deciding who should receive the heart transplant and who should not. Government policy in this area would free companies from blame, and they would have better relations with employees (Uchitelle, 1990: D2).

The kind of allocation decisions that will have to be made concerning how much our society will spend on organ transplants and intensive care units is being made plan by plan. We also allocate care by exclusion from the marketplace. The uninsured part of the population does not always get what it needs, especially in matters of routine care and regular checkups. They represent a special part of the population and will no doubt require some special planning to finance their care in the new age of managed care. Finally, as managed care spreads to the Medicare and Medicaid programs, new concerns will arise regarding quality and access to services, not just cost.

## REFERENCES

Broad, W. J. 1992. "Japan seen passing U.S. in research by industry." *New York Times* (February 25, 1992): C1, C10.

Cherkin, D. C., Grothaus, L., and Wagner, E. H. 1989. "The effect of office visit copayments on utilization in a health maintenance organization." *Medical Care* November: 1036–1045.

Eckholm, E. 1991. "Health benefits found to deter job switching." *New York Times* (September 26): A1, B12.

Freudenheim, M. 1990. "Business and health: Most want U.S. to pay the bill." *New York Times* (July 3): D2.

Freudenheim, M. 1991. "Health care a growing burden." *New York Times* (January 29): D1, D9.

Freudenheim, M. 1992. "Managed Care: Is It Effective?" *New York Times* (September 1): D2.

Gray, Bradford H. 1991. *The Profit Motive and Patient Care: The Changing Accountability of Doctors and Hospitals. A Twentieth Century Fund Report*. Cambridge, Mass.: Harvard University Press.

Kramon, G. 1989a. "Business and health: Controlling costs: One good sign." *New York Times* (April 18): D2.

Kramon, G. 1989b. "Business and health: Two companies cut medical costs." *New York Times* (November 7): D2.

Pallarito, K. 1995. "Execs: It's cool to be hot. Yet few have HMO skill in demand." *Crain's New York Business* (August 28): 32.

Salak, J. 1995. "Small companies flocking to managed-care option." *Crain's New York Business* (August 28): 31.

Schorr. A. L. 1990. "Job turnover—A problem with employer-based health care." *New England Journal of Medicine* (August 23): 543–545.

Shapiro, M. F., Ware, J. E., and Sherbourne, C. D. 1986. "Effects of cost sharing on seeking care for serious and minor symptoms." *Annals of Internal Medicine* 104, 2: 246–251.

Shellenbarger, S. 1990. "As HMO premiums soar, employers sour on the plans and check alternatives." *Wall Street Journal* (February 2): B1, B4.

Spragins, E. 1995. "Examining HMOs." *Bloomberg Personal* (October): 6–11.

Thurow, L. C. 1984. "Sounding Board: Learning to say no." *New England Journal of Medicine* 311 (December 13): 1569–1572.

Uchitelle, L. 1990. "Business scene: Seeking U.S. aid for health care." *New York Times* (May 21): D2.

# 3
## Medicaid Managed Care

The greatest concern we have is access to care, in particular specialty care. . . . It's the medical complexity and diversity of these children that make it hard to get them care in a managed care organization. It's like trying to put a square peg in a round hole when you try to fit these children into traditional health care systems.

—Julie Beckett, *Family Voices* (1995)

More than 35 million low-income Americans received health and long-term care through Medicaid financing in 1995. As the sole-source payer for the poorest of the poor, Medicaid, over a 30-year period, has created access to health care for many who would not be able to afford it. Prior to Medicaid and Medicare, the poor and the elderly had lower visit rates to doctors than those better off or younger. This is no longer true. Moreover, Medicaid has freed many families from the financial burden and social obligation of caring for the elderly or people with disabilities who cannot fully care for themselves by paying for various forms of long-term care. Consequently, the American nursing home industry is heavily dependent on Medicaid support. Without this form of financing, many facilities would not be able to pay their bills and would have to close, with the residents relocated elsewhere, most likely with relatives in the community. While some may argue, with much merit, that family care is better than nursing facilities, many opportunity costs would have to be borne if nursing facilities closed, with some middle-aged women having to leave the workforce to care for frail and declining relatives. In essence, Medicaid has supported the liberation of daughters from parent care, much as Head Start and day-care centers have enabled young mothers to go to work. The great secret of Medicaid is that it sustains new middle-class lifestyles. There is a need, however, to focus on why state-run Medicaid is moving its beneficiaries toward managed care at a rate that is even more rapid than is found in health plan benefits packages for the employed.

This chapter reviews briefly the history of Medicaid and why this uniquely American solution to the problem of how to pay for the care of the medically indigent emerged. This chapter also deals with the transformation of Medicaid acute care into a capitated payment system for health maintenance organizations. Changing the health-care environment for the poor has produced some disruption of services, reductions in services, and even fraudulent activities by providers in several states. However, researchers demonstrated some greater continuity of care, with stronger emphasis on prevention than was true in the past among providers serving the Medicaid-eligible population. Finally, we examine whether long-term care could work under capitation.

## ORIGINS AND STRUCTURE

While the employer-based insurance system provided a great deal of population coverage, by the 1950s it became evident that the poor elderly and women and children on public assistance could not gain access to health care because they could not pay for it. The Kerr–Mills Act was the model for Medicaid because it provided states with matching federal dollars to finance medical assistance for poor elderly Americans. When Medicaid replaced this program, it extended coverage to other impoverished groups, including people with disabilities and women and children supported under Aid to Families with Dependent Children (AFDC). Note that the incremental pattern of covering new beneficiaries was established long before our current health-care financing system was patched together.

Medicaid encouraged the development of medical services and access for poor people, often where none existed, through a complex transfer of revenues from the richer states to the poorer states. Federal and state dollars were matched according to a formula based on the average income in the state. Therefore, poorer states got more federal dollars than richer states. State responsibilities for the medically indigent were retained, along with obligations to take care of the severely mentally ill and mentally retarded populations, some of whom require 24-hour-a-day care. The federal dollars for this program were drawn out of general taxation revenues, unlike Medicare which was supported through payroll taxes and premiums charged to beneficiaries. Moreover, benefits in Medicare, mirroring Social Security pensions, were uniform across all states in recognition that retired people might migrate and need to have the same coverage wherever they went. In fact, portability of old age pensions and Medicare has created the foundation of a good life for the elderly in the United States.

Medicaid, in contrast, was a national program with state administration. Under Title XIX of the Social Security Act—the enabling legislation for Medicaid—federal standards established that in each participating state, eligible individuals were entitled to a basic set of medical and other health services. States could offer optional services as long as they maintained the basic federal package. Some large industrial states such as California, Ohio, and New York have been very generous in the kinds of services they will pay for. Less generous are the prairie states such as Idaho, Montana, and Wyoming. Optional services frequently covered are intermediate-care facilities for the mentally retarded, prescription drugs, dental services, podiatry, optometry, prosthetic devices, and eye care (Iglehart, 1993: 897).

States also administer the Medicaid program, exercising considerable latitude in determining eligibility for benefits and the amount of remuneration to providers. Eligibility varies widely from state to state, and some states can be very limiting as to who is covered. Less than half of the people who fall below the poverty line in the United States are financially eligible for Medicaid. In 1993 income eligibility ranged from a low of $1788 in Alabama for a family of three to up to $11,076 for the same-size family in Alaska. These low-end income cutoffs left many vulnerable and working-age people outside of the Medicaid safety net.

States also vary widely as to Medicaid reimbursement to providers. But in every state, rates for covered procedures for ambulatory care and *per diem* payments to hospitals for inpatients do not come close to what private insurance pays. Consequently, in every state there is cross-subsidization by private insurers of acute care for Medicaid beneficiaries as well as the uninsured who receive uncompensated care, largely from hospitals. Hospitals are compensated by formula from Medicaid for bearing what is called a disproportionate share of care for the medically indigent. Yet for voluntary hospitals that must provide Emergency Department services as well as admit Medicaid-eligible patients along with the uninsured, cross-subsidization is necessary to meet expenses. Ultimately, some of the cost is borne by employers who provide health-plan benefits or share the cost of such plans with employees.

An additional financial stress was added to Medicaid through efforts to protect children. In the 1980s, largely through the efforts of California congressman, Henry Waxman, coverage was extended beyond the traditional welfare population to pregnant women for prenatal services and all children under the age of 6 in families with incomes up to 133 percent of the federal poverty level. This program does make a difference: Significant improvements in access to care meant that poor sick children were receiving necessary medical care. A 10-year retrospective analysis of National Health Interview Surveys from 1982 to 1991 found that "Medicaid coverage increased utilization of illness-related care for low-income children to levels comparable to that of children in higher income families" (Gavin, 1996: 151).

Additional optional coverage was also made available to pay for pregnancy-related services for women with incomes up to 185 percent of poverty. Similar Medicaid coverage up to the age of 18 would now be available for all children born after 1983 and who were from families below the poverty line. States also made it somewhat easier for adults to become eligible for Medicaid as the economy increased the number of unemployed. As insurance expert Deborah J. Chollet notes, "Between 1989 and 1992, the number of people under age 65 who qualified for Medicaid coverage increased 38 percent, and then by another 9 percent between 1992 and 1993" (1996: 37). Now one out of every eight people in the United States below the age of 65 is covered by this form of public insurance, and within this group, one out of four children below the age of 18. As I discuss later in this chapter, some states have attempted creatively to extend Medicaid to the uninsured through conversion to managed care.

The increasing numbers on the Medicaid rolls did not reduce the number of uninsured in this country, with approximately 41 million uncovered by either public or private insurance. The rising costs of health care and, consequently, the cost of insurance, have led many employers to drop coverage for employees and their dependents. The problem of how to provide quality care at reasonable costs for the entire population did not disappear with the end of the health-care reform in 1994.

## RISING COSTS

The federal deficit shed new light on costs. The additional coverage of vulnerable populations through congressional authorization and working-age populations through downward mobility, the states extending optional services, and rising medical prices produced additional expenditures and brought Medicaid a great deal of new attention in Congress and state capitals as well. Medicaid costs started to rapidly outstrip increases due to medical inflation in the private sector and Medicare. This rise in costs far surpassed the increases of previous periods and caused concern about the financial viability of this key element in the country's social safety net.

The Medicaid population, because of its poverty, may be greater users of health-care services than those not eligible for Medicaid. Yet many ambulatory-care providers either refuse to see Medicaid patients because of low remuneration or limit the number of Medicaid patients in their panel so that they can generate more income seeing patients with other forms of insurance coverage. As a result of the combination of the severity of need and the lack of access to providers in the community, many individuals eligible for Medicaid use hospital clinics or overuse Emergency Departments. The limited access to primary-care physicians who can manage sick patients, in the opinion of some health-services experts, suggests that poor women and children will do better under some form of managed care that provides easy access to a regular source of care and the opportunity to learn good health practices.

While managed care may be good for poor women and children, states have adopted it mainly because it is seen as a way of reducing the costs of Medicaid. These new programs are cost-driven, but they will not have an enormous impact on state or federal Medicaid expenditures when all eligible women and children are enrolled in these health maintenance organizations. Although low-income families make up 75 percent of the Medicaid-eligible beneficiaries, they receive only 30 percent of the expenditures. This disproportionate distribution of resources results largely because, given their needs for nursing care and support services found in nursing facilities and intermediate-care facilities, the long-term care population is expensive to maintain. Predictably, state government has shown a great deal of interest in applying the lessons learned from acute managed care to long-term care.

Still, the idea of introducing managed care to the acute-care services for Medicaid beneficiaries does allow state health planners to follow a model found in the non-Medicaid sector of the population and the services they receive in either nonprofit or profit-making health maintenance organizations. By 1994, 23 percent of all Medicaid enrollees were in managed care arrangements. The Kaiser Commission on the Future of Medicaid reported in 1995 that "the most significant growth occurred between 1993 and 1994, when Medicaid managed care enrollment grew 63 percent, from 4.8 million beneficiaries to 7.8 million" (HCFA, 1994).

The reelection of Bill Clinton has been accompanied by a sharp reduction in the rise of Medicaid costs, as mentioned in the Introduction. This reduction of anticipated federal expenditures has promoted the idea of extending Medicaid benefits to poor and near-poor children who do not have insurance. To make this plan work, the states would have to contribute financially, as they do for all Medicaid recipients, and some states might not go along with this idea. In addition, in late 1996 there was also some discussion about helping to subsidize private health insurance for working people.

The full implications of these ideas need to be modeled to understand their impact. These two proposals need to be combined in such a way that they do not neutralize each other and prevent attaining the goal of extending coverage to the uninsured. As policy analyst and reporter Robert Pear (1996: A12) pointed out, the two proposals might produce the unintended consequence of having some states reduce Medicaid eligibility to take advantage of federal assistance with regard to the purchase of private health insurance. A review of the experiences of states that have attempted to extend private insurance through subsidy might reveal some interesting paradoxical outcomes.

## EXPERIENCE WITH MANAGED CARE

Despite this recent conversion to managed care, this kind of delivery system for Medicaid-eligible people is not as new as it seems. One state, Arizona, starting in 1982 with a waiver of the Medicaid regulations, operated the first and then only statewide prepaid Medicaid system. You might say that cost containment was its middle name. Designated the Arizona Health Care Cost Containment System (AHCCCS), it not only went from no state financing of indigent care to managed care but also included, through subsequent waivers, long-term care services for the elderly, the developmentally disabled, and the physically disabled (Fisher, 1994: 320).

Under AHCCCS, a monthly capitation fee covers each individual in a given contracting health plan. Adjustments are made in the rates based on extensive medical encounter and resource utilization data that help to place beneficiaries in different risk pools. In addition, health plans are able to purchase state-financed reinsurance to compensate for financially risky beneficiaries whose annual costs exceed $30,000.

Despite the strong emphasis on cost containment, no major deficits in medical care were found when the system was evaluated. Comparative studies with the conventional Medicaid program in New Mexico, a state with similar demographics to Arizona, found similarities in the quality of care in prepaid and fee-for-service medicine. In addition, a controlled study for the years 1989 and 1990 which reviewed 121,874 hospital patient discharges for 11 different conditions found few significant differences in utilization and mortality compared to patients with private insurance (Burns, Wholey, and Abeln, 1993). Some differences in utilization patterns were found among women who delivered babies in hospital, suggesting some underuse as well as overuse by Medicaid-supported patients.

Arizona was soon joined by most of the other states on the bandwagon to managed care as they created voluntary enrollment or local demonstration programs for HMOs. In 1994, 43 states reported financing the operation of at least one managed care program (HCFA, 1994). To operate this way, a state has to have HCFA approval through a waiver (1915b), which limits freedom of choice. The waiver allows states to require beneficiaries to choose a primary-care provider and continue with that provider for more than one month.

Some states used the 1915b Waiver as a way not only to lock in their Medicaid expenditures for the AFDC population but also to extend Medicaid eligibility to the near-poor or those with moderate incomes who have no health insurance. Sliding scales have been created for premiums as well as some other cost-sharing requirements. Hawaii, Oregon, Rhode Island, and Tennessee applied for permission to extend Medicaid benefits to people previously ineligible because of income. Unlike Arizona, all four of these more recent state-waiver plans allow individuals with disabilities to continue to see their providers, although some capitate the payments while others rely on fee-for-service remuneration. Like Arizona, having a large Medicaid pool makes it possible to negotiate favorable rates in contracts with health plans. The addition of previously uncovered individuals makes the state's bargaining position even more effective.

The extension of coverage to the uninsured who did not qualify previously for Medicaid because of their income is based on the idea of cost sharing with these new beneficiaries. However, the experience from Tennessee suggests that premiums and co-payments discourage the newly covered from staying with the program when renewal time comes. The near-poor do not find an income-adjusted premium appealing enough to stay with the plan.

Determining the real costs for HMOs requires careful scrutiny of the actual population that joins the health plan rather than for all the Medicaid-eligible population. When beneficiaries are given a choice between fee-for-service and HMO plans, and when plans can be selective, there can be overpayment to HMOs. This situation reflects the often noted fact that those individuals with serious chronic illnesses elect to stay out of HMOs—especially when it costs them nothing to see a physician in fee-for-service medicine. Those who join HMOs do not stay with their doctors because they are not as dependent since they rarely have chronic illnesses. The states, however, use data for the entire Medicaid population to do rate setting, thereby overrewarding HMOs through capitation, while the case mix for the HMOs does not include so many people in need of medical care. Indeed, some evidence exists that Medicaid bidders do not always take all eligible voluntary enrollees but often engage in the "cherry picking" or "cream skimming" that non-Medicaid HMOs have been accused of doing. West and his colleagues (1996) found that Baltimore-based HMOs serving Medicaid beneficiaries enrolled children with significantly lower utilization rates than children in the control population.

Additional implementation problems emerged with mandatory enrollment in Medicaid managed care plans. States and some municipalities that have fiscal responsibility for supporting Medicaid (as in New York State) have had to establish tough review criteria after some HMOs that held contracts with the states were viewed as not providing good care or went out of business when faced with the problem of actually having to provide care to thousands of poor people. In some places, recruitment was based on false claims to potential subscribers. State departments of health decided to slow down recruitment and make sure that bidders for contracts had the *capacity* to deliver the services they promised.

Proposals requested from bidders were required to address questions concerning how new members would be enrolled and oriented to the plan, the extent to which choice of primary-care physicians would be offered, what mechanisms were in place for changing doctors, as well as how quality assurance would be maintained, along with establishing a procedure for dealing with patient grievances. In addition, various other issues were addressed that would promote patient use of services, such as available transportation to doctors, or related to the qualifications of staff, including experience with high-risk populations.

Concern for quality also involved examining in the proposals how individuals with serious chronic conditions (e.g., asthma) would be identified and treated. A strong emphasis on health education was expected from bidders. Plans were expected to offer childbirth and parenting education, nutrition counseling, and smoking-cessation classes, along with immunizations.

Finally, all credentials for health-care providers with the plan were checked, along with the plan's record with voluntary Medicaid-managed care patients for any evidence of civil rights violations. Even a clean record, however, did not mean that the program was good at making users welcome. Important criteria related to access were evidence of wheelchair accommodation, location near the population to be served, 24-hour-a-day phone coverage, evening and weekend appointment hours, and a multilingual staff.

These reviews of bidders was based to some extent on some of the experiments with mandated managed care that occurred under special circumstances in several states in the early part of this decade. Originally conceived in 1987, southwest Brooklyn became the living laboratory for New York State's Medicaid managed care. The major concern was access to primary care for children in an area where few pediatricians were available and where children were often seen in hospital

Emergency Departments for conditions that could be treated elsewhere. This program enrolled over 30,000 Medicaid beneficiaries under the age of 21 in six different health maintenance organizations.

Several different types of plans were awarded contracts. The older nonprofit staff or group-based programs, because of their centralized locations, were better able to provide continuity of care than networks of physicians organized by for-profit corporations. Moreover, they were better at establishing procedures for educating enrollees about the appropriate use of emergency services and why members should restrict their use. According to the report of a New York City watchdog voluntary agency—the Citizens Committee for Children—part of their success comes from more experience with both operating an HMO and working with a low-income population. The longer parents were enrolled in an HMO, the more likely they were to follow recommended procedures before taking their children to the Emergency Department (Citizens Committee for Children, n.d.).

## COST SAVINGS

There is a strong need to determine whether managed care saves money for the states and the federal government, particularly as more and more states seek waivers and as Congress pushes the Health Care Financing Administration to create incentives for Medicare-eligible people to join HMOs. Two studies of efforts to introduce primary-care case management (PCCM) only in several states came up with inconclusive findings. Gatekeeping in these experiments was aimed at reducing inappropriate use of emergency services and specialty visits by increasing access to primary care. PCCM only pays a capitation fee or fee-for-service to a provider who takes on the responsibility of routine and regular care for a patient *without* any financial risk and absent of any effort to integrate services. Buchanan and her associates (1992) evaluated the organization and structure of 10 operational sites and the impact on service use and costs of randomly assigned and self-selected patients. Results differed strongly in New York and Florida. Hurley, Freund, and Paul (1993) examined the impact of PCCM in 25 programs in 16 states to determine whether gatekeeping of this kind reduced use of specialty care. When payments to primary-care providers were based on capitation, therefore introducing a financial risk for the provider, specialty care was not used as frequently as in fee-for-service PCCMs. As Hurley et al. note, "It is likely that substitution of primary for specialty care occurs in both arrangements" (p. 101).

The data from 130 studies collected and reviewed by the Kaiser Commission on the Future of Medicaid (Rowland et al., 1995) suggest a definite shift in types of services delivered, with greater use of primary-care providers and reduced use of specialists and Emergency Departments. Despite this complex study, no evidence exists that managed care reduces hospitalization, the number of physician visits per beneficiary, or the use of preventive services.

While it seems reasonable to predict that less use of specialists and Emergency Departments will reduce costs, there is mixed evidence to support this position; some studies even show no savings at all. Where studies do show savings, they range from 5 to 15 percent when compared to fee-for-service medicine. With primary-care providers doing more for patients than in the past, as financial incentives and the culture of managed care take over, we may see them both acting more cautiously than in the past when there is no support from specialists and hospitalizing patients or running more tests. At the same time, there is the danger that primary-care physicians may overlook or not treat conditions that may become more serious and require later hospitalization. Some anecdotal evidence from Tennessee shows that primary-care providers are now stretched to the limit because they are doing procedures that used to be performed by specialists. In addition, they spend a good deal of their time trying to find specialists who will accept the low fees available through the plan. One general internist, J. O. Patterson III of Memphis, admits that the procedures he handles could be performed better by those specialists trained to do them.

> It's a sometimes daunting responsibility to be entrusted with the care of these patients and to know you are not going to be able to offer state-of-the-art care for their problems. They may not be able to see the subspecialists who are more skilled in treating their ailments. (Brown, 1996: A6)

Concerned professionals such as James A. Blackman, the editor of *Pediatrics*, a widely read and respected professional journal, has written that

> The emergence of Medicaid managed care systems is particularly troubling. There are many stories of disrupted services, misleading information regarding choices of providers, and a lack of sensitivity to the feasibility or desirability of options. (1996: v)

Dr. Blackman recounts how a mother was inconveniently offered speech therapy for her preschool-aged child at a clinic 25 miles away, though with cab service provided.

The response of enrollees to Medicaid conversions to managed care is also mixed. Patients are most satisfied with Medicaid managed care when they can continue a relationship with a doctor from fee-for-service practice and follow her or him into the plan. Like all of us, Medicaid-eligible individuals want a physician who knows them well and can orchestrate their care.

Maintaining comprehensive and continuous care is not always possible even when beneficiaries have to select a regular source of care. A study of Philadelphia's medical assistance population that became part of the Hospital of the University of Pennsylvania's HMO found that 75 percent of billed services were not subject to the control of the "gatekeeper" in the form of a primary care provider (Hillman et. al., 1991).

While little is known about how special populations fare in Medicaid managed care, there is great concern that access to specialists will mean a reduction in the quality of care for individuals with serious chronic illness or disabilities. Articulating this concern has been a major goal of the Federal Maternal and Child Health Bureau. It has supported a number of policy studies that have raised questions about the extent to which quality care will be available in an age when plans are especially cost driven. Published in the journal *Pediatrics*, these papers raise serious questions about HMOs in general through discussions of the vulnerability of children with chronic illnesses, who constitute a surprisingly large portion of Medical-eligible children.

Access to care has become a central issue. Newacheck and his colleagues (1994) warn that cost considerations can create unacceptable situations for both parents and providers.

> If services are to be provided in the fee-for-service system, care must be taken to ensure that children are not "dumped" on outside providers to reduce expenses within the plan. In either case, out-of-plan services should be provided by recognized child health practitioners. Moreover, explicit contractual provisions must be made that describe how out-of-plan services will be provided and that delineate the plans' responsibilities for assuring children's access to specialty services and for coordinating such care with in-plan services. (p. 499)

The authors also raise questions about the capacity of a plan to serve this population, including:

- Is a multidisciplinary team of children's practitioners available?
- Are there linkages between Medicaid managed care plans

and existing public programs serving children with special needs (e.g., Title V Maternal and Child Health Block Grant Program)?

- Are there in place practice guidelines and performance standards, and capacity for monitoring compliance with them, for childhood chronic conditions?

- Are there written policies concerning grievance procedures?

- Are there written policies concerning access to care, including referrals to pediatric specialty care, and is information available about the qualifications of practitioners?

Still, one evaluation of Medicaid managed care in New York City found that managed care enrollees, compared to conventional Medicaid enrollees, had greater access to a usual source of care, more opportunity to see the same clinician at that location, and significantly shorter appointment and office waiting times. Managed care enrollees also reported higher levels of satisfaction (Sisk et al., 1996: 50).

While this study reinforces the belief that managed care provides greater access and continuity of care for Medicaid recipients, concerns also exist about the suitability of managed care for low-income children in general, and not just those with serious chronic illnesses. This is particularly the case because plans contracted with and supported by state Medicaid authorities are modeled after the plans that serve middle-class families. Hughes and his colleagues (1995) point out that "low-income children are more likely to experience a learning disability, and to have had a long-term emotional or behavioral problem" (p. 592). Given the harsher physical environment as well as greater family stress and hardship, this population needs more psychosocial support and care coordination than children from better off families. Unfortunately, HMOs do not traditionally make the linkages to social services required by families vulnerable to these risks.

## MEDICAID MANAGED CARE AND PEOPLE WITH DISABILITIES

Serving people with disabilities in Medicaid managed care programs has been attempted in 17 states. Yet only Arizona, Delaware, Oregon, Tennessee, Utah, and Virginia have required that beneficiaries with disabilities receive their medical care through capitated programs. Arizona, with 70,000 disabled in prepaid care programs, is the only state program with at least three years of experience.

A major concern of all these programs is how to set rates for people with disabilities when expenditures between disabilities and within categories of disability vary widely. Various methodologies and regulatory efforts have been generated to prevent health plans from avoiding Medicaid beneficiaries with complex medical problems and from sustaining enormous financial losses when they do take care of this population sector. The most common form, "reinsurance," is based on the states' sale of insurance that provides a guaranteed halt of the dollar loss to a plan caused by caring for enrollees with catastrophic expenses. Risk-adjustment formulas based on either prior experience with expenditures or on disease category have also been used, although each methodology has some serious flaws. Finally, another form of protection against severe loss to a plan is called a "risk corridor" arrangement. In this scheme, the plan and the state share losses but also provide a cap on how much money a plan can retain after paying medical and operating expenses for high-cost beneficiaries (United States General Accounting Office, 1996).

## WILL LONG-TERM CARE CAPITATE?

Once again, only Arizona has any extensive experience with managed long-term care for the Medicaid population. The six years in which capitated long-term care existed in the Roadrunner State marked a shift from no Medicaid involvement to complete managed care of all populations. The Arizona Long-Term Care System (ALTCS) integrates acute and long-term care services to its eligible beneficiaries. When compared to a control population in traditional programs in other states, participants have fewer hospital days, fewer procedures, and more evaluation and management services (McCall et al., 1996). The program pays for services for 20,000 enrollees. Approximately two-thirds are elderly and physically disabled, and one-third are mentally retarded or developmentally disabled. Prior to 1988, Arizona paid for some of these services, required localities with some state assistance to pay for others, or simply did not have the services available. Counties continue to provide matching payments for services for the elderly and physically disabled, whereas in the case of the mentally retarded or developmentally disabled, the state matches federal subsidies.

ALTCS has two administrative features. First, preadmission screening is rigorous, ensuring that only those truly in need of the supported levels of care get services. Second, acute and long-term care dollars are melded in a capitation payment, thereby providing an incentive to keep beneficiaries out of hospital and allowing for the substitution for skilled-nursing facilities and intermediate-care facilities with programs identified as home- and community-based services. Under yet another waiver from the Health Care Finance Administration, people with developmental disabilities are provided services that Medicaid traditionally did not pay because they were not considered to be medical in nature.

Made law as a part of the Omnibus Budget Reconciliation Act of 1981 (PL 97–35), the Home and Community-Based Services Waiver Program (section 2176) was conceived as a way of containing the increasing costs of institutional care paid for from federal revenues. The funding authority for this program came from amendments to the Social Security Act, wherein states could receive Medicaid matching funds to provide home- and community-based services to individuals who otherwise would receive care in a nursing home. The unique feature of this program was the authorization it gave state Medicaid to pay for clinically appropriate nonmedical services, including case management, habilitation services, homemaker services, personal care, and adult day care.

The original purpose of the home- and community-based waiver program was to dampen the demand for institutional care by making other, more affordable community-based services available to low-income individuals with chronic disabilities and illnesses. Under this waiver, the U.S. Department of Health and Human Services allows states to finance community services through Medicaid for people with developmental disabilities who would otherwise be in intermediate-care facilities (ICF) (Castellani, 1987). Designed to divert the flow of clients from the community into expensive ICF programs, by 1992 the home- and community-based waiver programs were operated in 48 states (Smith and Gettings, 1992). In 1991, $1.7 billion was spent on this program, with 65 percent of the total going for care of individuals with mental retardation (Miller, 1992). By 1995 all 50 states were participating in the waiver.

Although the Arizona program is based on capitation, it also features some cost containment features found in other states that do not capitate long-term care, including rate setting, intensive screening for eligibility, and case coordination. Most significantly, it has achieved service substitution by going directly to the home- and community-based services model, without ever developing an intermediate-care facility program. This means that it never really had to deal with an established set of providers concerned about protecting their programs and the higher rates they receive for care of this population.

Other innovations have come from grass-roots sources. A great deal of attention is directed toward Minnesota and its Long-Term Care Option Project (LTCOP), which was designed for elderly people who are eligible for both Medicare and Medicaid. Acute and long-term care services are integrated and "coordination is accomplished across provider type, settings, time and funding sources" (Minnesota Department of Human Services, 1995). Local by design, LTCOP plans operate as full-risk providers. Designated community-integrated service networks (CISNs), they may be formed by HMOs, insurers, hospitals, provider networks, local governments, or purchasers. These entities receive capitated funds from both Medicare and Medicaid at a rate adjusted for predicted expenditures for individuals who choose to receive their care through these programs. This financing stream is central to the program since medical costs for this population exceed that for any other long-term care population. However, to drive costs down requires care coordination. The formation of CISNs is an attempt to avoid duplication of services or utilization of a service that is simply available through a third-party payer rather than one that is appropriate to the patient's needs.

While all these approaches to cost containment have a great deal of merit, most of the savings realized by acute-care HMOs has been through favorable market conditions—the oversupply of doctors and hospital beds—which makes it favorable for payers to get deep discounts. There is no comparable surplus among long-term care providers. The field of long-term care does lend itself to service substitution, with home care replacing nursing facility placement and informal care networks pitching in to assist the frail elderly or developmentally disabled individuals with several functional deficits.

Some policy analysts worry that as state funding and block grants from the federal government for Medicaid continue to shrink, the work of long-term care will not only be based on replacement of skilled with less skilled providers, but also some, if not the entire, burden of care will once again be offloaded on daughters and parents. Furthermore, the long-term care field has developed based on the idea that consumers have choices to make with regard to services since much of this care is related to where they want to live and not just to who is going to give them their insulin. Much has been learned over the last 25 years about how to humanize care for vulnerable populations. Even the word "care" is rejected as being patronizing and has been replaced with the idea of services. With the current trend toward downsizing, consumer satisfaction has taken a back seat in the drive toward individual autonomy, and even customer choice may be stalled.

Ironically, the downsizing of government and its role in and initiating supporting innovative service arrangements means that we may soon long for the return of that supposed federal monolith that ideologues saw as a threat to individuality and choice. In actuality, the Department of Health and Human Services, the Social Security Administration, and the Department of Education, when generously funded by Congress, promoted many innovations in community services and the establishment of national standards. It is heartbreaking to see that the quality of life considerations and empowerment that have evolved as part of the home and community care movement may be sacrificed on the altar of cost containment.

Finally, the measures of quality that the National Committee on Quality Assurance is developing for Medicaid managed care focuses almost exclusively on services provided women and children. How can this methodology tell us anything about the quality of care for people with serious chronic illnesses and disabilities? Surely, HMOs are there for the sick as well as the healthy, and it is important to know how well they do in providing complex services for complex cases.

## REFERENCES

Beckett, Julie. 1995. *Family Voices*. 1.

Blackman, J. 1996. "From the editor." *Pediatrics* (October 3): iv–v.

Brown, D. 1996. "When specialists aren't the norm." *Washington Post* (June 10): A1, A6.

Buchanan, J. L., Leibowitz, A., Keesey, J., Mann, J., and Damberg, C. 1992. *Cost and Use of Capitated Medical Services: Evaluation of the Program for Prepaid Managed Health Care*. Santa Monica, Calif.: Rand R-4225-HCFA.

Burns, L. R., Wholey, D. R., and Abeln, Marty O. 1993. "Hospital utilization and mortality levels for patients in the Arizona Health Care Cost Containment System." *Inquiry* 30: 142–156.

Castellani, P. 1987. *The Political Economy of Developmental Disabilities*. Baltimore, Md.: Paul H. Brookes.

Chollet, D. J. 1996. "Redefining private insurance in a changing market structure." Pp. 33–62 in Stuart H. Altman and Uwe E. Reinhardt, eds. *Strategic Choices for a Changing Health Care System*. Chicago: Health Administration Press.

Citizens Committee for Children (n.d.). "Finding a way through the labyrinth: Medicaid managed care for children in southwest Brooklyn." Unpublished paper. New York: Citizens Committee for Children.

Fisher, R. S. 1994. "Medicaid managed care: The next generation?" *Academic Medicine* 69: 317–322.

Gavin, N. I. 1996. "The impact of Medicaid on children's health service use: A ten-year retrospective analysis." Abstract from the 13th annual meeting of the Association of Health Services Research, Atlanta, Georgia, June 9–11.

Health Care Financing Administration, Office of Managed Care. 1994. *Medicaid Managed Care Enrollment Report Summary Statistics as of June 30, 1994*. Washington, D.C.: U.S. Department of Health and Human Services.

Hillman, A. L., Goldfarb, N., Eisenberg, J. M., and Kelley, M. A. 1991. "An academic medical center's experience with mandatory managed care for Medicaid recipients." *Academic Medicine* 66: 134–138.

Hughes, D. C., Newacheck, P. W., Stoddard, J. J., and Halfon, N. 1995. "Medicaid managed care: Can it work for children?" *Pediatrics* 95: 591–594.

Hurley, R. E., Freund, D. A., and Paul, J. E. 1993. *Managed Care in Medicaid: Lessons for Policy and Program Design.* Ann Arbor, Mich.: Health Administration Press.

Iglehart, J. K. 1993. "Health policy report: The American health care system: Medicaid." *New England Journal of Medicine* 328 (March 25): 896–900.

McCall, N., Wrightson, C. W., Korb, J., Crane, M., Weissert, W., and Wilkin, J. 1996. "The Arizona Long-term care system: Six years of experience integrating acute and long-term care in a capitated Medicaid program." Abstract from the 13th annual meeting of the Association of Health Services Research, Atlanta, Georgia, June 9–11.

Miller, N. A. 1992. "Medicaid 2176 home and community-based waivers: The first ten years." *Health Affairs* 11 (Winter): 162–171.

Minnesota Department of Human Services. 1995. "Updated summary: Long term care options project." Unpublished paper. Minneapolis: Minnesota Department of Human Services.

Newacheck, P. W., Hughes, D. C., Stoddard, J. J., and Halfon, N. 1994. "Children with chronic illnesses and Medicaid managed care." *Pediatrics* 94: 497–500.

Pear, R. 1996. "Clinton now looking at incremental approach to health-care reform." *New York Times* (November 11): A1, A12.

Rowland, D., Rosenbaum, S., Simon, L., and Chait, E. 1995. *Medicaid and Managed Care: Lessons from the Literature.* Washington, D.C.: Kaiser Commission on the Future of Managed Care.

Sisk, J. E., Gorman, S. A., Reisinger, A. L., Glied, S. A., Dumouchel, W. H., and Hynes, M. M. 1996. "Evaluation of Medicaid managed care: Satisfaction, access, and use." *Journal of the American Medical Association* 276 (July 3): 50–55.

Smith, G. A., and Gettings, R. N. 1992. *Medicaid Funded Home and Community-Based Waiver Services for People with Disabilities.* Alexandria, Va.: National Association of State Mental Retardation Program Directors, Inc.

United States General Accounting Office. 1996. *Medicaid Managed Care: Serving the Disabled Challenges State Programs.* Washington, D.C.: GAO/HEHS 96–136.

West, D. W., Stuart, M. E., Duggan, A. K., and Deangelis, C. D. 1996. "Evidence for selective health maintenance organization enrollment among children and adolescents covered by Medicaid." *Archives of Pediatric and Adolescent Medicine* 150: 503–507.

# 4
# Healthy and Unhealthy People at the HMO

> [I]t is critical to find a payment system that mixes the prospective and retrospective components in a manner that will create incentives to economize while limiting profits stemming from undertreatment.
> —Richard G. Frank, Thomas G. McGuire, and Joseph Newhouse,
> *Health Affairs* (1995)

Washington, despite the optimism of 1993–1994, produced no great health-care reform. The following two years produced a law making insurance coverage portable from job to job, with the Kassebaum–Kennedy bill barely making it because it was mired in politically unacceptable amendments designed to kill it. Almost like a stealth bomber, the managed care forces overtook fee-for-service medicine and introduced capitation. The private health insurance industry got into the act as the most heavily capitalized of the developed HMOs and managed care products. The irony is that the Clinton plan that the nation rejected because of its complexity has arrived by the back door. The now defunct 1342-page Health Security Act produced by a health-care reform Task Force, composed largely of health-care policy experts and assembled in Washington in 1993, relied heavily on a service-delivery model that expected many Americans to voluntarily join health maintenance organizations (HMOs). Despite the demise of this detailed legislative plan for reorganizing and refinancing the American health-care delivery system, and five years before the millennium, a new age of managed care has arrived.

It is no exaggeration to say that we are in a new age of health services. Competition has forced the private insurance sector, a business that once avoided controlling services, to move so far in the direction of managed care that it has become increasingly more difficult to find a policy that does not include some cost-containing components. These features were added to make these plans attractive pricewise to corporate benefits officers, and as a result, they sold briskly in the early 1990s. Conducted in 1993, a national survey of almost 2000 employers found that over half were in managed care plans, up from 29 percent in a similar polling in 1988 (Gabel et al., 1994). Straight indemnity insurance policies are becoming increasingly harder to find in the benefits packages at America's corporations. And, of course, the need to restrain public spending has produced Medicaid managed care. Given these trends, it is time to ask about the impact of financing on health care. Does less service amount to greater value? In other words, are HMO members getting good medical care, and are they being kept as well as their fellow Americans with indemnity insurance?

HMOs started both to feed on and catch up to the current American concern about taking care of one's self as the best kind of insurance. Wellness became something to be sold, not just something from the Sunday supplements or part of the soft news found nightly on television. HMOs have marched to the wellness tune to sell both to employers and employees. Discounted memberships in fitness clubs are part of the sales pitch, attracting the well and discouraging the chronically ill, people with disabilities, or those who don't look good in spandex. But HMOs say it is in their interest, not just the consumer's, to keep enrollees fit. In theory, HMOs remain solvent by keeping people well and permitting early detection of disease, thereby minimizing overall expenses required for hospitalization and specialty care. Moreover, no perverse financial incentives are offered providers to deliver unnecessary services, including referrals to expensive specialists or orders of inappropriate high-technology, but often unnecessary, diagnostic testing.

## THE MEDICAL ADVANTAGES OF PREPAID HEALTH CARE

Health-service researchers and policy analysts are engaged in strenuous debates over the virtues and deficits of managed care. Without question, the HMO system lowers financial barriers for members by establishing modest visit payments, thereby making direct contact with a physician or surrogate easier than for self-paying (i.e., uninsured), Medicaid-eligible, or for those covered by private indemnification insurance. Many HMOs, particularly the nonprofits, have 24-hour access to a primary-care physician or a nurse. For some medical emergencies, for example, an acute appendicitis, research indicates that the incidence of a ruptured appendix, a condition that can be life threatening, is lowest among HMO enrollees (Braveman et al., 1994).

In discussing this study, Arnold Relman, former editor of the authoritative *New England Journal of Medicine*, cautions us to be careful in interpreting these results. Superiority in treating an acute appendicitis does not mean that HMOs are necessarily a superior form of organizing medical services for *all* contingencies.

> Acute appendicitis may be almost unique in this respect, or it may be one of many conditions in which greater availability of primary care and easier access to medical attention in emergencies confer substantial health benefits on members of HMOs as compared with patients covered by indemnity insurance. We simply do not know. (Relman, 1994: 471)

Still, despite Relman's questioning of whether one study validates the merits of managed care, other studies have shown easy access to care to have enormous benefits. Prevention through early detection of some cancers in their initial stages was found to occur more frequently for HMO members than for those Medicare patients in the fee-for-service system (Riley et al., 1994). Performance of screening services is part of the HMO approach to health-care delivery. Some HMOs also promote the use of such services through educational programs for members. The strongest impact of HMOs on early detection was found among the data collection sites where there were large and more established HMOs.

The quality of care at HMOs is based not only on early detection but also on ease of access to prevention in the form of immunizations, acquisition of good nutritional habits, and programs to encourage smoking cessation. The AAHP publication, *Healthplan Magazine*, reinforces this approach through a philosophy of care that stresses a baseline physical examination, prevention, and early identification of disease. Through this approach, in *Healthplan Magazine* author Thomas N. Bethell highlighted the success of HMOs in identifying life-threatening conditions previously unknown to the patient.

In these areas of health maintenance, HMOs have been consistently ahead of traditional fee-for-service doctors. But what about referrals for specialty care, particularly expensive surgical procedures? After all, opting not to do the bypass operation helps preserve the financial resources of the HMO as a business. Perhaps being slow to refer to a thoracic surgeon may preserve the HMO's well-being at the expense of the patient's health or longevity.

How do HMOs do in comparison to fee-for-service medicine? A study in Detroit of patients who had coronary artery bypass graft (CABG) surgery found that there were no delays in referral for surgery for HMO patients with coronary heart disease and that outcomes were approximately the same for the two concurrent groups of patients (Paone et al., 1995). Yet a study in one location may not represent HMO practices everywhere. HMOs may get deep discounts for this procedure in the Motor City—a metropolitan area with such an excess capacity of CABG surgical units and surgeons that some Canadian provinces allow some patients with coronary heart disease to cross the border and be treated in these settings rather than build such units at Canadian hospitals.

What about access to less dramatic interventions? Critics of managed care sometimes see other services as vulnerable to the cost-saving goals of HMOs. These concerns have led some investigators to the conclusion that home care would be suboptimal when an HMO had a risk-based contract with Medicare. However, Adams, Kramer, and Wilson (1995) found similar outcome scores when HMO patients were compared to fee-for-service patients.

Similar results were found when managed care programs for people with affective disorders were matched with fee-for-service psychiatric services. A British review article on studies in the United States did not find that cost containment meant lower quality of services for depressed elderly inpatients (Wells, 1995). Nor were patient functioning and well-being profiles along 12 domains different in three distinct programs self-selected by participants (Stewart et al., 1993).

These results may be reassuring when questions of quality of care are raised. But most studies that compared outcomes between fee-for-service and HMO plans only followed patients for one year. Over a four-year period of observation, a more recent prospective investigation of 2235 patients, conducted as part of the Medical Outcomes Study, found worse physical outcomes in HMOs than fee-for-service system (Ware et al., 1996). People with hypertension, non-insulin-dependent diabetes mellitus, recent acute myocardial infarction, congestive heart failure, and depressive disorder were followed from 1986 to 1990. Those chronically ill patients who were elderly and poor had worse physical health outcomes in HMOs than in fee-for-service systems. Patients with these characteristics were more than twice as likely to decline in health in an HMO than in a fee-for-service plan. Mental health outcomes were inconclusive and may be related to different HMO sites.

The results in the Medical Outcomes Study for high-risk patients suggest that the quality of care in HMOs deserves a close look beyond the averages for all patients. There is also concern that many serious conditions can be ignored in HMO primary-care settings. During the early 1990s, many newspaper and evening news stories revealed false negatives—overlooking the presence of disease—and misdiagnoses in HMOs, and attributed them to the practice of cost-conscious medicine, for example, where access to Magnetic Resonance Imaging equipment is restricted. Tales were also carried about delays in getting appointments for this kind of testing or in seeing specialists. How HMOs care for sick people is the crucial test for this form of medical organization and financing, as it is for any other. The outcomes of medical events related to sick people constitute meaningful measures of quality for HMOs, the equivalent of launching a rocket to the moon for NASA.

The last 10 years have been a learning experience for patients and their physicians; quality as well as mediocre care, despite limits on access to specialists, is available in HMOs. In truth, the quality of medical practice within and outside of HMOs is virtually the same. The old canard that only doctors who could not make it on their own joined HMOs has been put to rest, even by the American Medical Association. Patients were quick to realize that quality was not limited to fee-for-service medicine. What doctors in private practice were finding out was that families with routine needs for medical care were deserting them in droves. During the 1980s and 1990s, HMO membership grew steadily as cost-conscious consumers acted to make their health-care expenses more predictable and as a variety of financial arrangements were made with providers, using many different forms of compensation. With no deductibles and minor co-payments for visits to the doctor, young families with children found many advantages in having virtually unlimited access to primary care through pediatricians or advanced practice nurses called pediatric nurse practitioners. The 1986 National Health Interview Survey found that 13 percent of all children under the age of 18 belonged to HMOs, including approximately 400,000 children with serious chronic health conditions.

## MANAGED CARE AND CHILDREN WITH SPECIAL HEALTH-CARE NEEDS

The current expert assessment on the quality and quantity of research on Medicaid managed care, or the experiences of other families with special needs children in health maintenance organizations, is that their knowledge of children with special health-care problems is woefully inadequate (McManus, Fox, and Leibowitz, 1993: 4). With more and more families in health insurance programs that have managed care components, it is important to ensure the quality and access to care for children with special health-care needs.

With quality, access, and cost the major concerns during this period of transformation, some vulnerable groups are alarmed at the private and public trends toward managed care. Advocacy groups for people with disabilities view cost containment as a dangerous way to provide care to all, perhaps at the expense of those with the greatest needs. The outcry in 1991 about possible rationing in the Oregon Medicaid plan was at that time seen as evidence of this concern. In anticipation of some of the major financially driven components of health-care reform, Andrew Batavia, executive director of the federal National Council on Disability, concluded that "cost containment provisions that focus on the provider, such as global budgeting and managed competition, will adversely affect disabled people if providers do not have adequate incentives to meet these people's needs" (1993: 41).

It is also possible to suggest the alternative view—based on the health maintenance organization model of service delivery—that coordinated and comprehensive care and preventive services will be more readily available to children with disabilities than through traditional fee-for-service medicine. In particular, the fragmentation of the specialty health-care delivery system could be overcome through case or care coordination. Finally, designed to reduce the need for hospitalization, the HMO emphasis on routine preventive care and ease of access to ambulatory care would seem to enable the child with special needs to have a more normal lifestyle, as well as reduce the likelihood of unnecessary utilization.

Access to care has been a consistent problem for families of children with special needs. The goals of any health-care reform should be consistent with the objectives of a national disability policy that ensures that all people with disabilities, including children, have access to the services they need, without compromising quality or creating enormous financial burdens for their families. Families of children with special health-care needs "must have access to a health care system that ensures a comprehensive array of services, including health, rehabilitation, personal assistance and support services across all service categories and sites" (Batavia, 1993: 44). Moreover, this system should be efficient; should not discriminate against people with disabilities; should permit individualized services plans; and should distribute costs fairly so that families with members who are disabled are not disproportionately burdened.

In the current era of health-care privatization, families that include children with special needs represent a vulnerable population. While such groups have been identified by the United States surgeon general and other leading health-care experts as requiring "family-centered community-based services" for their children with special needs, we currently do not know if this is what they seek, or get, in the way of services. Therefore, Medicaid reformers and those state officials with oversight authority on private health plans need to be guided by the evidence found in states where the bulk of the population has direct experience with HMOs.

The experiences which Medicaid-eligible families of children with developmental disabilities have had with cost-conscious HMOs may provide some answers to questions about how to provide good care for this vulnerable population. This idea of medical care organization has been applied to keeping Medicaid expenditures down. The state governments' efforts to save money are not without problems. Buchanan (1992), for example, reported that special needs populations sometimes find it difficult to identify a plan that offers providers with experience dealing with the clients' special health conditions. Little is known about whether Medicaid-enrolled children with special health-care needs and their families who require *collateral services* are able to receive such services from managed care providers. Moreover, how can the quality of care standards for these children be assured? (Fox and McManus, 1992: 51).

HMOs may not always meet parent or professional expectations precisely because children with serious chronic illnesses or developmental disabilities are more likely to need specialty care more frequently than other children. These illnesses and disabilities require periodic visits to a variety of specialists to determine whether a therapeutic regimen should be continued, altered, or discontinued. Moreover, they may also need access to such related services as speech therapy, physical therapy, mental health services, and appliances. Such interventions or treatments may not be available through knowledgeable pediatric specialists employed by the HMOs, but may be otherwise available in the community through public or privately operated clinics in which are found specialists or groups of providers not affiliated with an HMO.

Concerned observers and policy experts have argued that HMOs that attempt to ration care can restrict access to specialty care, and that a capitated-rate structure does, in fact, encourage this. Thus, families may have greater access to care but not to the right kind that will meet their special needs. Yet it is not known whether the financing and organization of HMOs plans actually affect health outcomes for children with special needs.

Finally, many insurance policies, and HMOs as well, do not cover the full range of services that children or adults with handicapping conditions need. HMOs typically cover only short-term inpatient rehabilitation and often do not pay for wheelchairs or other assistive devices (Batavia, 1989). Medicaid has traditionally been more comprehensive than most private insurance plans in covering direct and collateral services for children with disabilities and their families. Certainly, traditional Medicaid coverage may be advantageous for families of children who require a disproportionate share of services. But without systematically collected information from states with the greatest use of HMOs for Medicaid patients, it is hard to know how to plan and prevent limitations of access to services for low-income families or children with serious chronic illnesses or severe developmental disabilities.

Professionals as well as parents are concerned about the problem of access. The American Academy of Pediatrics Child Health Financing Report has noted the concern that underservice may be an outcome of health-care reform. Yet what is known about managed care for children does not provide much of a guideline for establishing a major reorganization of health-care services.

> ... the impact of managed care on children with special needs and on adolescents has never been studied. What little is known regarding the public and private managed care experience and young children derived mainly from studies on Medicaid recipients conducted over 10 years ago. No comparable large-scale studies have been conducted on managed care in the private sector. Moreover, the newer models of managed care (e.g., IPAs and PPOs), which are likely to form the basis of managed competition, have not been studied at all. (McManus, Fox, and Leibowitz, 1993: 3)

HMOs may provide comprehensive acute care for healthy children but not give benefits for children who have ongoing problems. A close examination of the benefits available for children with six chronic diseases and developmental disabilities reveals gaps in coverage in both traditional indemnification policies and HMOs. Horwitz and Stein (1990), respectively, a public health specialist and a nationally recognized pediatrician with expertise on the delivery of medical services to children, examined six of the largest indemnity insurers and the six largest HMOs registered in the state of Connecticut. After acquiring information on the benefits structure of each plan, along with built-in mechanisms for restricting or limiting health services, six case vignettes with medical conditions that varied in urgency, intensity of service need, and chronicity were created. These conditions included a broken clavicle, a case of multiple trauma that included a fractured femur and internal injuries, an episode of otitis media, chronic otitis media with a question of language delay, spina bifida, and juvenile diabetes. Thus, two cases involved developmental disabilities as well as serious chronic illness.

The cases were usually presented to the account executives who negotiated the benefit plan or to a customer claims representative from the insurers. Given that certain medical services and equipment were medically appropriate, these vignettes were designed to determine what the insurers and the HMOs would pay for or provide.

The results were that "both health maintenance organizations and traditional indemnity insurers tended to have restrictions for specific services needed by children with chronic illnesses, such as medical equipment and mental health services. *Case managers in both systems tend to control expenditures rather than to coordinate care*" (italics added) (Horwitz and Stein, 1990: 581). While calling for "the more extensive evaluation of the generalizability of these findings (p. 581)," Horwitz and Stein also observe that there is little information about the experiences of families in regions with large, long-standing HMOs (p. 586). Therefore, any study of the impact of managed care on children with special health-care needs should go beyond a single state or metropolitan area.

A major concern of health-service researchers is that HMOs might reduce access to care for children with chronic conditions. Yet contrary to this view, a single-site study of visit levels for children with allergies whose families switched from traditional indemnification (Blue Cross) to an independent practice association, found that prior to the switch, the children had 41 percent fewer well-child care visits than did other Blue Cross allergy patients. Enrollment in the IPA encouraged preventive and acute-care visits for these children with minor illnesses (Szilagyi et al., 1992). (It is also possible that parents reduced visits during the year prior to conversion to the IPA plan, knowing that certain well-child visits would be covered during the following year, and that visits might level off in subsequent years.) To what extent do these findings hold for children with developmental disabilities?

Nationally collected data on the subject of managed care and children with special health-care needs are often limited to summaries of the literature and in-depth interviews with professionals. While useful in providing some data on consumer satisfaction, the experts often are not fully familiar with how HMOs serving Medicaid patients are organized and deliver services. Following interviews with experts from state Children with Special Health Needs agencies, the members of the American Academy of Pediatrics Committee on Children with Disabilities, and parent organizations, Fox et al. (1990: 116) reported that large HMOs were viewed as better staffed to provide appropriate medical care than smaller HMOs. Expert opinion held that nonmedical services such as physical, occupational, and speech therapies were very limited within HMOs. However, no consensus existed on the question of access to proper equipment and supplies. In the absence of systematically collected data, the authors of this study conclude that questions remain as to whether the quality of case management services meets the needs of families of special needs children (Fox et al., 1990: 121).

With indications that health-care marketing and private benefits management are moving toward wholesale reliance on managed care systems, reports on consumer experiences and satisfaction with HMOs for families that have special needs children are important but rare dispatches. Evidence remains limited to one region, without taking into account variability in the mix of insurance coverage. In a survey of five HMOs serving state employees in two urban counties in Wisconsin, Karlson, Sumi, and Braucht (1990: iv) found that "for many families, financing certain health care services which no insurance plan will cover will be a more difficult task than choosing between the HMO and a fee-for-service plan." High levels of satisfaction were based on good relationships with physicians and other providers, overall low costs, and reduced paperwork. Some parents had difficulties with HMOs in "determining which specialty services were covered, obtaining and maintaining referral authorization for specialized services, and a lack of choice of specialty providers" (Karlson, Sumi, and Braucht, 1990: iv).

Central to satisfaction with services in the Wisconsin study was the establishment of a good relationship with the primary-care physician. Referrals for specialty care were not a problem under this circumstance. The HMOs studied did not seem to ration care; nor did they have an established policy on standards of care for each serious chronic illness or disability. Future expansion of HMOs would need to take into account parent views as to what constitutes "good" care and to what extent this matches up to professionally developed standards (e.g., number of regular visits during a year to a specialty care source, at which time appropriate therapeutic services are being provided).

Managed care systems function as passive as well as active constraints upon referrals. Drawn from a sample of American Academy of Pediatrics' fellows, pediatricians surveyed about their experiences with referral barriers in managed care systems reported somewhat less referral of patients in these systems than in traditional pay systems. Moreover, more than 20 percent of the sample of pediatricians with patients in managed care systems experienced the denial of at least one referral to subspecialist care and 10 percent inpatient care in the year under review. Pediatricians experienced more barriers from preferred provider organizations than from HMOs (Cartland and Yudkowsky, 1992: 183).

A common way to develop process measures of the quality of care is to establish periodicity schedules for children of different ages. One countywide study of a Medicaid case management demonstration project on primary care found that capitation payment, untied to the delivery of services, did not reduce access to primary care (Hohlen et al., 1990). The authors also believed that future research on capitation programs needs to examine the process of service delivery for children with acute and chronic conditions. This must necessarily include the difficult task of developing consensus among experts as to what constitutes appropriate care for chronic illnesses affecting children. (Hohlen et al., 1990: 68)

During the summer of 1993, I conducted a focus group interview with five mothers of offspring with developmental disabilities, with ages ranging from the mid-thirties to under five. A focus group interview is an excellent way to find out about the challenges of enrolling special needs populations in HMOs. My purpose was to examine how parents of children with developmental disabilities choose health-care plans and to evaluate their experiences in them. In this effort, I adapted the *focus-group interview technique* to the study of consumer experiences with health services. This technique, used by social scientists and market researchers for 50 years (Merton and Kendall, 1944), has helped researchers learn at close range about how decisions and preferences develop. In this approach, questioning follows a funnel approach, moving from the general to the specific. To maximize the investigators' sensitivity to the participants' concerns, the "questions vary in response to the character and requirements of each individual or group exchange" (Goldman and McDonald, 1987: 10). This session produced some interesting findings concerning experiences with HMOs, particularly for parents of children who had reached their adult years.

Two important findings emerged from this group interview. First, half the questions were *anticipated* and did not have to be asked because the parents were as concerned with the issues behind the questions as we were. This indicated that the questions touched an important aspect of their lives. Second, self-advocacy was an important skill in gaining access to services covered by the contract with a staffed HMO but might not be directly available.

Following are some excerpts from this focus-group interview. In response to a question concerning how one mother became involved with the HMO, a mother suggests the importance of continuity.

We were covered by this HMO before my children with disabilities were born. With J., I realized something was wrong with his eyes. The HMO pediatrician could not figure it out. I got a referral to a specialist at Beth Israel. The HMO paid. We found out J. had congenital glaucoma. Over the years, one thing the HMO was not able to do was to give me specialists. For orthopedics, there is nobody . . . for seizures, there is nobody. They are there for pediatrics. Anything that

I need them to write up, I have to dictate. They themselves
are not trained to deal with our children. I had a pediatrician
for all these years. When J. got sick recently as an adult and
had to go to an ICU, I had to lose my pediatrician. I am
altogether lost now because I have an internist who has
never dealt with the handicapped. You asked why we stay
with this HMO. I still have a pediatrician treating my 35
year old son. Even after I stopped working for the City I
picked it up to keep contact with her. They also made a referral to the Hospital for Special Surgery, and this HMO
paid. I had to fight with them for each payment over a number of years, but they paid for the orthopedist and for the
appliances.

Typically, the responses to questions showed great variability when
specialists were requested by parents.

### DID YOU EVER GIVE THE NAME OF A SPECIALIST TO WHOM YOU WANTED THE CHILD TO BE REFERRED?

*Respondent 1*: We are limited to HMO doctors.

*Respondent 2*: My doctor did not hesitate to recommend
an outside specialist to me that they paid for.

*Respondent 3*: They wouldn't pay for a pulmonologist if
they had one on their list.

### DID YOU EVER HAVE DIFFICULTY GETTING ACCESS TO A NEEDED SERVICE?

*Respondent 4*: The HMO centers used to have physical
therapists around, but they never had people trained to
deal with children with developmental disabilities.

*Respondent 5*: In my case I wanted my son to get physical therapy at the HMO. I was told that he can't get
physical therapy because he was born with the condition. But they would give some one who got hurt on the
job PT. If HMO is the thing of the future, parents have
to be taught how to advocate with the staff. They have
to be advocates for their kids.

If children with special health-care needs are enrolled in large numbers in HMOs or other managed care plans, their parents will not only
have to fight for their services, but these plans may also lose their
competitive advantages. The selection process for HMOs and other
managed care plans has excluded many individuals with serious

chronic illnesses for two reasons. First, fewer of them are in the work-force and cannot gain access to plans that are largely tied to contracts with employers. People in the workforce tend to be younger and health-ier than the rest of the population. Given these characteristics, they bring fewer complicated medical problems to service providers. Second, whether we are considering adults or children, where serious chronic illness is concerned, patients or their guardians are very reluctant to change providers who may not be part of the various managed care networks and plans that exist. What advice can a benefits officer at a corporation give to an employee whose family can share in the savings afforded by participation in an HMO but who will be forced to give up an ongoing relationship with a pediatric cardiologist who has been treating since birth a child with a congenital heart defect? Clearly, many families will stick with what they know rather than take a chance on the unknown. Still, even those families that select a policy that per-mits unrestricted access to doctors who receive fee-for-service payments may find themselves subject to managed care provisions such as prior authorization for surgical procedures if the insurance company will pay for the procedure.

## LIMITS TO THE SAVINGS ENGENDERED BY MANAGED CARE

Managed care and HMOs are here to stay. The oversupply of doctors in the United States has made network membership or fixed-salary arrangements attractive to physicians who a few years ago would not think of joining them. HMOs use fewer physicians per every 1000 pa-tients than does fee-for-service medicine. Moreover, these prepaid plans select and hold on to physicians who can work under rules, not order up a great deal of testing, provide preventive medicine, and use hospitalization less frequently than other physicians. Some of the cur-rent proposed federal legislation would require HMOs that create pre-ferred provider organizations or independent practice associations, two basic designations for networks of doctors, to sign up any state-licensed physician who wished to participate in the network and accepted fees established by the HMO. If selectivity is eliminated, then it will be harder for HMOs to establish a uniform practice style that limits ex-penditures. In addition, in September 1994, the American Medical As-sociation produced and televised advertising, wherein its president, a surgeon, argues against managed care and the restriction of physician autonomy. Despite these protests, health care today is undergoing ma-jor organizational and financial restructuring—even without universal coverage or the elimination of denial of insurance because of preexisting conditions. Much of this transformation of our medical organization and hospitals was initially in reaction to the Clintons' health-care reform effort. During the deliberations of the national Task Force, under the direction of Hillary Rodham Clinton, the large insurance companies and major providers realized that the recommended reforms would be built on greater use of HMOs and managed care programs. Spurred on by this information, in 1993 the investors brought the industry further along the path of reining in doctors as the major source of inefficient use of health-care resources. The public rationale was that HMOs and managed care would shrink the waste in the system. However, the evidence on which this premise was based was somewhat suspect.

With the country increasingly moving toward managed care and HMO membership, the savings initially noted in the comparisons of costs when HMOs are compared with managed care plans, or straight indemnification, start to become less dramatic. A 1994 Congressional Budget Office (CBO) assessment of the effects of managed care on costs of service delivery supported the view that HMOs do save money but that their patient population is typically healthier than patients receiving care in fee-for-service (FFS) medicine. As more and more people join HMOs, the enrolled populations will begin to look more like the general population, including more sick people. This memorandum also finds that many of the studies comparing HMO costs to fee-for-service medicine compared insurance plans that had no managed care components, a luxury that few policies permit today. Therefore, the relative advantage of HMOs is decreasing.

> Recent nationally representative evidence (for 1989) indicates that the most effective HMOs can reduce use of services by about 12 percent compared with unmanaged care, or by about 9 percent compared with the FFS sector. When the performance of current HMOs (plans with varying levels of effectiveness is considered), evidence indicates that they reduce use of services by an average of about 7 percent compared with unmanaged care, and by an average of about 4 percent compared with the FFS sector. (CBO, 1994: v)

The review of studies conducted by the CBO also found that good HMO management could generate low-cost care, building on the independent practice association model as well as the staffed-model HMO. Making careful physician selection, improving access to and sharing of information among the participating physicians, putting providers at financial risk for cost overruns, and being a major source of each participating provider's patient panel are factors that keep costs down.

Some concerns remain about how to measure the comparative ad-

vantage of different approaches to paying the doctor to determine overall costs. Most comparisons of costs that examine prepaid versus
fee-for-service health care use the premium paid by the policyholder as
the basis for analysis. Although policies with deductible and co
payment features allow analysts to estimate out-of-pocket costs to subscribers, it is not very clear whether enrollees in HMOs bear medical
expenses outside of the HMOs, perhaps when they cannot get authorization or approval for procedures they strongly believe they need.

In a larger sense, every cost-shifting effort helps to destabilize our
health-care delivery system. Some health-care policy experts and economists find that the growth of managed care has led to a great deal of
cost-shifting as less and less is covered by policies (Freudenheim, 1994:
A17). The consumer has become one of the payers, albeit a somewhat
hapless player, in this game of trying to keep your costs down. For the
uninsured, sometimes decisions have to be made concerning purchasing prescription medications or some other necessity.

With regard to determining who pays for hospital costs, a more consistent bearer of the burdens of cost shed by HMOs has been all other
third-party payers. This may be one reason why HMOs can save money.
A managed care organization in a local area can negotiate a substantial
discount with a hospital for its subscribers. While the HMO may pay
for an HMO patient at a low rate, the hospital does not simply absorb
the cost. It is passed on to third-party payers that do not have the
advantages produced by contracts guaranteeing a certain volume of
patients per year. In addition, Medicare and Medicaid also pay hospitals at a lower rate than indemnity policies. Hospitals are willing to
extend these discounts because their bed census, often at 50 percent,
is so low that many are threatened with closing if they cannot generate
revenues. Hospital administrators worry about the future because currently only 38 percent of all privately insured people in the United
States are in traditional indemnification policies, the source of largesse
in the cost-shifting game. But the game is going to run out of "fat cat"
players before the end of the millennium.

The newly enacted Kassebaum–Kennedy bill, designed to create continuity of coverage, may make it easier for workers to accept new jobs
because they will not have to wait a year for coverage to begin for preexisting conditions. When these companies are forced to initiate premium increases, consumers will be driven to seek other kinds of plans.
Fewer third-party payers will be around to whom costs can be shifted,
and new financial arrangements will have to be made to keep the hospital system going.

Numerous financial arrangements have also been suggested to prevent HMOs from dumping high-risk cases or underserving this
population, leading to their disenrolling. The subject of rate-setting

capitation payments is employed or proposed as a means of compensating for greater use of services. It is an attempt to be fair to those health plans that take on their responsibilities fairly and receive bad risks. But how can the basis of the adverse risk be established?

Using data from Maryland and Minnesota, five leading models—a demographic model, ambulatory-care groups, ambulatory diagnostic groups, diagnostic cost groups and payment amounts for capitated systems—were tested for children with chronic conditions. No model was useful in predicting expenditures for these at-risk children (Fowler and Anderson, 1996).

Fowles and her colleagues (1996) attempted to compare the performance of different health status measures for risk-adjusting capitation rates. To collect data on total expenditures, a sample of 18–64 year olds (n=825) and a sample of those over 65 (n=955) at a Minnesota network-model HMO were followed during the year in which their health status was measured and the following year. Both self-reported health status and diagnoses predicted future expenditures twice as well as demographics. The authors concluded that without risk adjustment, capitation rates would either overpay or underpay. It would also be useful to see whether the same or greater amounts of service are delivered with risk adjustment than without it.

Physicians, consumers, and health-policy analysts have voiced concern that managed care may lead to less access to specialists with experience in dealing with serious chronic illness and disability. As a result, the Robert Wood Johnson Foundation, a leader in funding innovative projects in health care and in framing issues related to access, quality, and cost, has launched a chronic care initiatives program. In the mid-1990s, grants were awarded to various HMOs and academic medical centers, often as partners, in order to create solutions for some of the problems raised by depending so heavily on primary care for the bulk of medical services. Two examples demonstrate the kinds of innovations being attempted. First, a managed care college is being replicated at the Henry Ford Health System in Detroit to provide continuing education for primary-care clinicians as a means of increasing their capacity to care for selected chronic conditions. Second, the Group Health Cooperative of Puget Sound in Seattle is developing, evaluating, and disseminating information about how to provide "managed" primary care to patients with chronic conditions. A chronic care clinic will see frail elderly patients every few months for a half-day session, focusing on patient assessment, patient/family education, and provider/patient interaction. Between visits, midlevel health practitioners will monitor patient compliance to the care plan and arrange followup visits through frequent telephone contact.

Finally, the growth of HMOs also means that more primary-care providers and fewer specialists will be needed, creating new disruptions in the ranks of the medical profession. Current projections by health-care planners call for an expansion of primary-care providers so that by the year 2000, physician distribution will approximate the 50–50 split between specialists and generalists that exists in Canada and other countries with universal health-care coverage. This projection is based on greater access to primary care of the currently uninsured and underinsured and greater expansion of HMOs and other managed care programs. However, physician-supply projections indicate that even with 50 percent of medical school graduates entering generalist prac-tices, it would take until the year 2040 to achieve this kind of balance between specialists and generalists.

There is also an intriguing possibility that, with an expanded use of HMOs, the demand for *both* primary-care and specialty physicians will be reduced, especially if malpractice reform also takes place. Kindig and his associates (1993), though guarded in their willingness to ex-trapolate to the national supply, hint that HMOs may be able to deliver services with a ratio of three generalists to every specialist. "Staff and group model plans use about 130 full-time physicians per 100,000 en-rollees, of which 73% (95/100,000) are generalists. Of full- and part-time physicians combined, 49% are generalists" (Kindig, 1993: 1070). These ratios fall far short of the AMA and Association of Medical Col-leges recommended standards of 191 physicians per 100,000 popula-tion. Whereas in the past HMOs tended to attract healthy young families, a population that utilizes little medical care, the future will see a different mix, requiring perhaps more specialists than in the past. In the years to come more and more members of the medical profession will look back to a golden age of autonomy and substantial incomes.

## REFERENCES

Adams, C. E., Kramer, S., and Wilson, M. 1995. "Home health quality out-comes. Fee-for-service versus health maintenance organization enroll-ees." *Journal of Nursing Administration* 25 (11): 39–45.

Batavia, A. I. 1989. *The Payers of Medical Rehabilitation: Eligibility, Coverage and Payment Policies.* Washington, D.C.: National Association of Reha-bilitation Facilities.

Batavia, A. I. 1993. "Health care reform and people with disabilities." *Health Affairs* (Spring): 40–57.

Braveman, P., Schaaf, V. M., Egerter, S., Bennett, T., and Schecter, W. 1994. "Insurance-related differences in the risk of ruptured appendix." *New England Journal of Medicine* 331: 444–449.

Buchanan, J. L., et al., 1992. "HMOs for Medicaid: The road to financial inde-pendence is often poorly paved." *Journal of Health Politics, Policy and Law* 17 (Spring): 71–96.

Cartland, J. D., and Yudkowsky, B. K. 1992. "Barriers to pediatric referral in managed care systems." *Pediatrics* 89 (February): 183–192.

Congressional Budget Office (CBO) Memorandum. 1994. *Effects of Managed Care: An Update.* Washington, D.C.

Fowler, E. J., and Anderson, G. F. 1996. "Capitation adjustment for pediatric populations." *Pediatrics* 98 (July): 10–17.

Fowles, J. B., Weiner, J. P., Knutson, D., Fowler, E., Tucker, A. M., and Ireland, M. 1996. "Taking health status into account when setting capitation rates." *Journal of the American Medical Association* 276 (October 23/30): 1316–1321.

Fox, H. B., and McManus, M. A. 1992. *Medicaid Managed Care Arrangements and Their Impact on Children and Adolescents: A Briefing Report.* Washington, D.C.: Child and Adolescent Health Policy Center.

Fox, H. B., Wicks, L. B., Kelly, R. W., and Greaney, A. 1990. *An Examination of HMO Polices Affecting Children with Special Needs.* Washington, D.C.: Fox Health Policy Consultants.

Frank, R. G., McGuire, T. G., and Newhouse, J. 1995. "Risk contracts in managed mental health care." *Health Affairs* (Fall): 50–64.

Freudenheim, M. 1994. "Many economists say managed health care is no cure-all for soaring medical costs." *New York Times* (September 6, 1994): A1, A17.

Gabel, J., Liston, D., Jensen, G., and Marsteller, J. 1994. "The health insurance picture in 1993: Some rare good news." *Health Affairs* 1, 13 (Spring): 327–336.

Goldman, A. E., and McDonald, S. S. 1987. *The Group Depth Interview: Principles and Practice.* Englewood Cliffs, N.J.: Prentice Hall.

Hohlen, M. M., Manheim, L. M., Fleming, G. V., Davidson, S. M., Yudkowsky, B. K., Werner, S. M., and Wheatley, G. M. 1990. "Access to office-based physicians under capitation reimbursement and Medicaid case management: Findings from the Children's Medicaid Program." *Medical Care* 28 (January): 59–68.

Horwitz, S. M., and Stein, R. E. K. 1990. "Health maintenance organizations vs indemnity insurance for children with chronic illness: Trading gaps in coverage." *American Journal of Diseases of Children* 144 (May): 581–586.

Karlson, T. A., Sumi, M. D., and Braucht, S. A. 1990. *The Impact of Health Maintenance Organizations on Accessibility, Satisfaction and Cost of Health Care for Children with Special Needs.* Madison, Wis.: Center for Health Systems Research and Analysis.

Kindig, D. A., Cultice, J. M., and Mullan, F. 1993. "The elusive generalist physician: Can we reach a 50% goal?" *Journal of the American Medical Association* 270, 9 (September 1): 1069–1073.

McManus, M., Fox, H., and Leibowitz, A. 1993. "What we know about managed care for children." *American Academy of Pediatrics Child Health Financing Report* 10 (Spring): 3–4.

Merton, R. K., and Kendall, P. L. 1944. "The focused interview." *American Journal of Sociology* 6 (May): 541–557.

Paone, G., Higgins, R. S., Spencer, T., and Silverman, N. A. 1995. "Enrollment in the Health Alliance Plan HMO is not an independent risk factor for coronary artery bypass graft surgery." *Circulation* 92 (9 Supplement): 1169–1172.

Relman, A. S. 1994. "Medical insurance and health: What about managed care?" *New England Journal of Medicine* 331, 7. 471 172.

Riley, G. F., Potosky, A. L., Lubitz, J. D., and Brown, M. L. 1994. "Stage of cancer diagnosis for Medicare HMO and fee-for-service enrollees." *American Journal of Public Health* 84, 10: 1598–1604.

Stewart A. L., Sherbourne C. D., Wells, K. B., Burnam, M. A., Hays, R. D., and Ware, J. E., Jr. 1993. "Do depressed patients in different treatment settings have different levels of well-being and functioning?" *Journal of Consulting and Clinical Psychology* 61, 5: 849–857.

Szilagyi, P., Roghmann, K. J., Foye, H. R., and others. 1992. "Increased ambulatory utilization in IPA plans among children receiving hyposensitization therapy." *Inquiry* 29 (Winter): 467–475.

Ware, J. E., Bayliss, M. S., Rogers, W. H., Kosinski, M., and Tarlov, A. R. 1996. "Differences in 4-year health outcomes for elderly and poor, chronically ill patients treated in HMO and Fee-for-Service systems." *Journal of the American Medical Association* (October 2): 1039–1047.

Wells, K. B. 1995. "Cost containment and mental health outcomes: Experiences from US studies." *British Journal of Psychiatry—Supplement* 27 (April): 43–51.

# 5
## How HMOs Assure Quality

The challenge for health plans is to re-engineer the business so the product they are selling can be evaluated on a quality basis as opposed to a price basis.

—Ed Keaney, Volpe, Welty and Company
(Freudenheim, 1996)

The purchasers of HMO products are generally the benefits officers for large corporations or government agencies with many employees. Their major concern is the cost of the plan when considering which plans to choose for employees (Freudenheim, 1996: D5). Service to employees is also an important consideration, but the quality of care has not been of great concern when deciding whether to stay with a plan or enter into a contract with a new HMO or other kind of managed care organization. Because so many health plans exist in metropolitan regions, producing keen competition, purchasers of these services may leave after one or two years when they find a better price elsewhere. Slowly, buyers of health plans have shown an increasing concern about how good these HMOs are in delivering services, particularly when it comes to keeping people well.

Predictably, quality may make the difference in the purchaser's decision making when cost is basically the same. This lesson has not been lost on the sellers. Eve A. Kerr and her associates (1996) created a questionnaire to find out what kind of quality assurance programs capitated physician groups had implemented and to determine whether they emphasized the monitoring of overuse compared with underuse and improvement of preventive services rather than chronic disease care. The setting was a large network-model HMO in California, with

133 contracting physician groups. Ninety-four groups responded, representing 2.9 million covered lives.

The longer the physician group was in existence, the higher the profitability, and the more capitation penetrated their markets, the more likely the emphasis on quality assurance. The group's quality assurance programs monitored procedures subject to overuse, such as caesarean delivery and angioplasty rates, more than procedures subject to underuse, such as childhood immunization and performance of retinal examinations for diabetics. More effort was found in identifying underuse of preventive services than in followup services for people with chronic diseases. Enrollees were sent reminders for preventive services but not as frequently for chronic disease followups.

Preventive activities are generally cost-effective and offset later expenditures, but they cannot be equated with all of health care. As people age, they become subject to chronic diseases, most of which can be managed with appropriate followup. While it is more difficult to measure the quality of chronic disease care than immunization rates, the overall effort to do so remains low. With such a strong emphasis on certain measures, focusing on prevention and early detection of disease, physician groups and other managed care delivery systems may concentrate their service delivery in these areas, neglecting other parts of health care. To answer the critics of managed care, it may be useful to redefine the scope of quality assurance to include processes and outcomes that are difficult to measure.

Some movement has been made nationally in that direction. The American Association of Health Plans, the rapidly growing trade association, has spawned a quasi-independent organization that has generated complex review and evaluation standards to certify local or regional HMOs. Named the National Committee on Quality Assurance (NCQA), this organization has become the major source of information about the quality of care in HMOs.

Many HMOs, however, have made in-house efforts to collect data on their physicians' performance. For advertising purposes, plans may also participate in other quality assurance and consumer satisfaction studies. These efforts take time away from other tasks and are essentially duplicative. Parenthetically, if health-care reform was successful, one standardized instrument would have served to make sure that consumers and purchasers had the information needed to make decisions.

The development of quality assurance instruments is not a new idea. In the 1970s, the Health Care Finance Administration developed utilization review and established peer auditing to ensure good care for Medicare patients. In addition, in the same decade, a creation of the American Hospital Association, the Joint Commission of Accreditation of Hospitals, sought to guarantee the monitoring of quality of care in hospitals, and when indicated, efforts were make to improve clinical performance.

Today, the intense competition among plans has resulted in voluntary national efforts to establish baseline comparisons between health plans. NCQA has led the quest to establish valid and reliable indicators of plan performance and health outcomes. The availability of measuring tools also promotes interest in creating "Report Cards" for HMOs, with greater interest in establishing quality benchmarks than in the past. The pressure is increasing to learn about how well a plan does in treating diseases such as diabetes or glaucoma.

These results are recognized as critical to success in the managed care industry. The executives who run HMOs are concerned about making profits, but that is not their sole preoccupation. Good marketing, as well as good management, requires information about how well a health plan does and about what kinds of patients are served. To make money, an HMO has to attract and hold on to subscribers as well as use resources efficiently. Organizing a health plan in a particular locality is built on planning, information, and a generalized positive attitude toward the enterprise. Finding out whether one is getting good value involves analyzing the conditions under which care is delivered, performing interventions and preventive activities that are medically appropriate, and getting good results—as measured best in improvement in health or performance of the activities of daily living.

A program of good quality generates good results. It is based on the most valid knowledge about what works and what doesn't. An up-to-date physician does not continue to prescribe medicines that have been demonstrated to be ineffective or dangerous. In other words, a good delivery system makes strategic use of systematically collected information to obtain the most desired health outcomes. Sometimes the least expensive path to good outcomes is as good as the most expensive. Although some inexpensive medications to treat cardiac problems produced by the blockage of arteries have worked quite well, less is not always more. Some expensive drug therapies are superior to less expensive ones, and not all patients respond to inexpensive products. This knowledge is gained through carefully controlled studies and the accumulation of epidemiological data collected on populations over long time periods.

Not all knowledge comes from rigorously performed studies. Administrative data are also useful in determining whether resources are used efficiently. Traditionally, information collection has been part of the management style of both nonprofit and for-profit HMOs. Their management information services divisions have always collected a great deal of administrative data on how efficiently their providers use resources or whether some primary-care providers have disproportionately high turnover or complaint rates. These activities generally fall under the heading of *quality assessment*, which the Institute of Medicine (1990) defines as "the act of measuring quality of care, of detecting problems of quality, or of finding examples of good performance."

What is new and interesting is the extent to which data are used to reassure the public, government officials, and leaders in medicine that the use of managed care will not mean second-rate care for enrollees. Meeting the NCQA criterion, which its public information releases in a tone of self-congratulation sometimes call "the gold standard," represents an effort to remain free of regulation and to reassure a skeptical public that HMO medicine is as good as any medicine currently available. This is done in several tried and true ways, although there are limits to the measures they use.

Less common than quality assessment is the Institute of Medicine's own "gold standard" for review—*quality assurance*. This standard applies to activities beyond assessment, extending not only to identifying the problem but also verification, isolation of what can be corrected, initiation of interventions or corrections, and continuous monitoring to ensure that identified problems no longer exist. Furthermore, it seeks to make certain that no unintended negative consequences have surfaced during the correction process.

To understand the elements of a program designed to assess and assure quality, we need to examine how HMOs are constructed. The most important premise is that managed care be built on selectivity. It makes sense to the HMO planners to establish a health plan with the best doctors available and to retain them so that patients will get the best quality care possible. Good physicians will also need to receive the appropriate administrative and allied health-care supports for them to function well. Patients will need access to these providers and information on how to use the plan. For those patients who do not speak English, it will be useful to make translators available or to hire providers who speak foreign languages, for example, performing physical examinations in the patient's language. Those in charge of reviewing the quality of care determine how one health plan performs in comparison with another based on the structure of services that is in place.

Determining whether a plan meets expectations is a matter of reviewing the credentials of the providers and selecting not only those who are licensed but also those who have kept up with their fields of specialization. Being "board-certified" means in medical parlance that physicians have voluntarily taken a comprehensive test established by the specialty organization to which they belong and have passed that test. This test usually combines written and oral questions. The organizations that promote these examinations are sometimes called "academies" or "colleges" to indicate that they are scholarly in nature and are not just businesses set up to protect the material interests of the profession. Two such organizations are the American Academy of Pediatrics and the American College of Surgeons. After board-certification, the physicians may become fellows in one of those organizations, which signifies that they have accomplished something and that the additional abbreviations after the M.D. represent certification. HMO managers who are putting together a physician network or filling positions in a staffed-model program call this "credentialing."

HMO managers take the task of credentialing very seriously because of the prior aspersions cast on doctors who worked in HMOs or were paid a salary rather than a fee-for service remuneration. Historically, the American Medical Association, state medical associations, and leaders of county medical societies were contemptuous of HMO doctors, considering them failures who could not survive in private practice and who needed the security of salaries. But while keeping up with one's field is admirable, no hard evidence exists that board-certified physicians produce better outcomes than those without certification.

Today, some still are convinced of the superiority of the physician who works outside of the HMO system, although it is very hard to support the statement that HMO doctors are inferior to those who work outside health plans. Many doctors belong to several plans at once, which makes for all kinds of new relationships between colleagues who may never have met. Where once a surgeon received referrals only from primary-care doctors whom they knew, they now receive authorization forms for consultations from M.D.s they have never even heard of and certainly never met. Therefore, the idea of credentialing, though a selling-point to recruit enrollees, also reassures providers that they can trust the referrals they get and the subspecialists to whom they refer.

Establishing that the appropriate structure is in place for health-care delivery only means that the stage is set for good care. Measures of performance also occur in the field. These measures consist of simple or detailed examinations of standardized kinds of activities that assure the prevention of disease (e.g., immunizations) or testing for the presence of disease on a regular basis (e.g., doing a Pap smear). In addition, there are ways to determine whether good care is delivered when disease is present. Children, for example, often get painful middle ear infections (otitis media). There are standardized treatment procedures for this condition, and a process measure used to evaluate pediatric practice is whether those procedures are followed once the condition is identified. Clinical practice guidelines are becoming more and more important as resources become scarcer and as efficiency becomes a recognized value in health-care delivery.

Perhaps the best measure of quality is the result of an intervention. These so-called outcomes refer to making people well enough so that they can resume their normal activities. When a child with an ear infection receives an antibiotic promptly and is able to return to school quickly, missing fewer days than a child who is not treated in the same fashion, this is an indication that the medical intervention works or works better when done sooner than later. Outcomes are the most desirable measures of quality. They can be studied rigorously to determine which kinds of procedures work best or which providers get the best results. Medical outcomes studies can also tell us which patients respond best to the same intervention.

Outcomes are the broad measures of health status we have come to expect from public health sources (Donabedian, 1988). These measures include survival, longevity, functioning, and physical comfort, to name some of the more objective ones. Subjective measures, such as perceived well-being and consumer satisfaction, are used when objective measures are not available or take too long to determine (Starfield, 1992; Stewart and Ware, 1992).

There is no more graphic example of outcome measures than the death rates of patients who undergo heart surgery. Cardiac artery bypass graft (CABG) surgery has been reviewed very closely to determine whether some surgeons have greater success than others in keeping patients alive. These studies of mortality attempt to control for the patient's degree of impairment so that fair comparisons are possible. Some surgeons, perhaps even the very best, attract the sickest cardiac patients for whom the prognosis can be very poor. Biostatisticians adjust the risk associated with each patient so that there is a kind of level playing ground on which thoracic surgeons can compete. They have also discovered that the more operations performed, the better the success rate, suggesting that in complex tasks repetition remains a definite advantage. Some of these studies have also led to the discovery that those surgeons with the greatest success rates (i.e., capacity to keep their patients alive) do prepare the patient differently than surgeons with lower rates of success.

In some states, Pennsylvania, for example, these investigations of CABG have set a limit on who can perform bypass surgery. With the closing of some operating rooms and the restriction of this type of surgery to the certified, the mortality rate has gone down. In addition, the sharing of knowledge about preparatory procedures among the remaining approved surgeons has also improved outcomes.

The quality assurance teams established by NAQA have attempted to perform all three of these measures—structure, process, and outcome. Every HMO that volunteers for review must complete detailed forms to receive accreditation, identifying who and what they have available to deliver services. In addition, these health plans also are encouraged to cooperate in an additional data-gathering effort with an instrument called HEDIS—the Health Plan Employer Data and Information Set. Now in its third generation, this instrument consists of eight domains that seek to assess the quality of each plan. The previous version of HEDIS rated 330 health plans. The current version is built on this experience, as well as suggestions from various interested parties. These domains are

- Effectiveness of care
- Access/availability of care
- Satisfaction with the experience of care
- Health plan stability
- Use of services
- Cost of care
- Informed health-care choices
- Health plan descriptive information

New items are being tested to determine whether they can be used on a large scale. A substantial number of these new items relate to the effectiveness of care domain, and some are oriented to public health. These items include screening for the sexually transmitted disease chlamydia and determining the number of people in the plan who smoke and who have quit smoking. Other new items are related directly to followup of abnormal test results, patient compliance with treatment, or patient management both within and outside of hospitals when serious chronic disease is presented.

This approach has a number of flaws, mainly because it focuses on what is most easily measured. A number of biases are inherent in what is essentially a performance or process evaluation of managed care organizations. The developers of HEDIS readily admit that more of the reviews of effective care are based on the use of preventive interventions, for example, immunizations for children or the use of standardized tests, performed on people at the age when certain diseases usually have their onset. Usually, medical experts strongly recommend this kind of testing (e.g., mammography).

In response to criticism that followed earlier versions of HEDIS, a more strenuous attempt is being made to determine whether proper procedures were followed in treating people with serious and life-threatening diseases such as congestive heart failure. Although these diseases are chosen to some extent because large numbers of individuals contract them, more strategic reasons are behind this choice. Some of these procedures hold for all individuals who have this disease, and others are seen as necessary when information suggests that the patient is deteriorating or is at risk of decline if nothing further is done. Such measures are deliberately included because there is evidence that taking action at such times does make a difference in patient outcomes.

There is also a glaring absence of measures related to conditions that are rare or of low prevalence in the population. The originators of HEDIS reason that low-prevalence conditions or diseases do not provide a sufficient number of cases to satisfy the so-called power requirements of statistical tests needed to determine whether differences between plans are not due to chance. Serious chronic conditions (e.g., diabetes) that affect large numbers of people generate enough cases in each plan to make comparisons across plans possible and even comparisons among patients within plans. Alternatively, rare conditions such as cystic fibrosis, which affect only one out every 10,000 Americans, do not appear in sufficient numbers, even in the rare plan with 1 million members in a given region, to make powerful comparisons possible.

Access to care is as important as the effectiveness of care, especially if a person has a serious chronic illness or disability. HEDIS attempts to deal with the frequent criticism of managed care that enrollees do not get the care they need. When HMOs rely on primary-care providers to perform gatekeeping functions, patient dissatisfaction or disappointment in not getting to see a specialist may be expressed. A measure on whether consumers feel they experienced delays in getting care or a referral to a specialist is currently being evaluated for inclusion in a future reporting set.

For people with a serious chronic illness or disability, it is just as important that the primary-care provider have some experience taking care of people with special needs. If none of the primary-care providers in a plan is able to determine whether a person with spina bifida is deteriorating because none has had experience caring for this sector of the population, then easy access in the form of being able to get an appointment within a week after calling may not be meaningful. The process of credentialing should include a systematic effort to contract with and train at least some primary-care physicians or midlevel practitioners who can identify these warning signs for people with neurologic or orthopedic impairments. Of course, if a plan wishes to exclude such enrollees, they can make a deliberate effort to avoid hiring or contracting with such providers precisely because they might attract expensive and difficult consumers with multiple problems. The delivery of quality services to chronically ill or disabled individuals at this point in time in the evolution of HMOs will not be rewarded. The conscientious HMO may only attract more expensive cases, without landing any more of the healthy population whose capitation could offset the cost of delivery of complex and frequent services to those in greater need.

Plans need to provide data on disenrollment to HEDIS. Such information could help determine overall satisfaction rates for a particular HMO and also identify whether those with serious chronic illnesses or disabilities disenroll at a disproportionately higher rate than the healthy.

Such information should be made available to potential purchasers of the services of this plan and to current or future enrollees as well. HEDIS does look at whether a plan informs members about how the plan works. While this is required reporting, the specifications of HEDIS 3.0 (the third generation of HEDIS) do not indicate that it will provide a "drill down" capacity, as is found on the Internet, for individuals with special health-care needs. This capacity shows if any special features can help them learn how to use the plan more effectively. In other words, more information is available upon request that is tailored to the special concerns and interests of those with ongoing health problems.

Descriptive information on how the plan selects physicians, what policies exist on preauthorization of services, and how the plan monitors and manages care for serious illness is part of the final domain in HEDIS. This domain provides detailed information on the plan's structure, staffing, rules, and management philosophy. Under the subject of care management, a required measure is the approach taken in managing serious cases. As is stated in HEDIS 3.0 (1996: 49),

> Case management is the process of identifying patients at risk for costly care and developing ways to deliver quality care to these individuals. Each plan has its own methods of deciding which cases require case management, and creating services or programs for ongoing disease management and education.

Clearly, this is an important tool designed to help patients get better or to adapt to chronic conditions. But is it not important to determine whether the purpose of case management in a particular plan is to improve patient functioning, thereby demonstrating the effectiveness of care, or to conserve costly resources? While the two goals—effective care and resource management—are not mutually exclusive, sometimes the two clash. Reporting on the conditions under which this happens in case management, better expressed as care coordination, makes it possible to determine what specific services become involved in so-called judgment call decision making and which plans tend to experience more or fewer of these clashes. Given this track record, potential enrollees can be advised of what fate is in store for them, and plans can be rated as to how well they perform when care is vitally required.

Case management can orchestrate a variety of interventions, not all of them strictly medical. Some plans may make available a wide range of rehabilitation therapies to assist a patient following a stroke. Other plans may be very restrictive and reduce the possibility of delivering effective care. If HMOs are to deliver better care than fee-for-service medicine, then case management becomes crucial to patients' needs, regardless of cost.

Plans that seriously fall behind the middle of the pack of all the HMOs may raise important questions as to the management of these plans and even the quality of the medicine practiced. More precise distinctions may be very hard to achieve without creating misinformation for the public and regulatory agencies (Epstein, 1995: 59).

In certain areas, HMOs can rightfully pride themselves on being able to produce greater benefits than fee-for-service medicine. Ease of access to primary care should produce a definite advantage in achieving early diagnoses of some life-threatening diseases, yet little process or outcome differences are reported in one investigation. A comparative study of the quality of care for colorectal cancer conducted at the University of Texas Health Science Center, for example, found no differences between fee-for-service and HMO cases in terms of duration of symptoms before diagnosis and several other parameters related to diagnosis, including rates of survival. Other differences such as time from detection to treatment had no effect on survival rates after adjusting for age and stage of diagnosis (Vernon et al., 1992).

Similar results were found in a one-year study of 5295 people with rheumatoid arthritis cared for in fee-for service and prepaid group practice settings (Yelin, Criswell, and Feigenbaum, 1996). For 11 years, the study team followed 341 people. On either an annual or a long-term basis, the quality of health care appeared similar for patients seen in either setting, with no differences shown in the number of office visits, outpatient surgeries, hospital admissions, and painful joints.

While HEDIS 3.0 included a domain on satisfaction with the experience of care which should be sensitive to some of the access issues raised in the preceding discussion of case management, no specific questions were addressed to consumers about how people with chronic illnesses or disabilities fare in HMOs. Fortunately, a national survey, the Consumer Assessment of Health Plans, is planning to include a substantial set of questions on what health-plan enrollees with such conditions experience with regard to access to specialists and therapies. Comprised of six sections, this instrument does not limit itself to HMO members but also reaches consumers with indemnity insurance and those covered by a preferred provider organization. The survey questions focus on the last medical visit and the consumer's experience during the last six months (Department of Health Policy, Harvard Medical School, 1996).

This survey seeks to gain information about utilization, access, and degree of satisfaction with services. Another goal is to determine whether various problems identified by consumers are attributed to health plans or providers. Thus, gaining access to needed care or approval or referrals or preauthorization by the plan is a central concern of the researchers who as of the summer of 1996 were field testing their instruments. Some specific questions are as follows.

- In the last six months, have you had any problems arranging to see a specialist who has adequate experience evaluating and treating a specific condition you have?

- In the last six months, has your health insurance plan refused to approve or pay for any medical care or tests that you thought you needed?

- In the last six months, have you postponed or gone without medical care or medicine that you needed because your health insurance didn't cover it?

It is possible to compare similar populations in fee-for-service and capitation to determine whether they have equal access to care. Mauldon and colleagues (1994) compared the extent to which children with special needs in a single HMO over a two-month period have comparable access to acute-care visits and checkups as in the fee-for-service system. Few differences in use of the health services were found. However, given the fact that major disabling conditions were present in this sample of 1685 children, a more crucial comparison would have been to see whether access to specialty care was similar or different. After all, few pediatric providers can on their own manage conditions such as blindness, diabetes, cerebral palsy, mental retardation, and amputations.

This raises another important consideration. In a highly cost-conscious service environment, some observers have suggested that there may be some reluctance to introduce new treatment modalities when they are not part of the standard benefit package or are likely to increase expenses (Ireys, Grason, and Guyer, 1996). Similarly, lockstep protocols for providers do not always allow for the use of clinical judgment, especially when it costs the plan money (Herbert, 1996).

Concern about the quality of care in HMOs has also become the responsibility of the Health Care Financing Administration (HCFA), with almost 10 percent of Medicare beneficiaries in health plans and 74 percent having access to at least one managed care plan. Enrollments were growing in 1995 at 75,000 a month, and future efforts to reduce the cost of the Medicare program will be built on encouraging senior citizens to choose HMOs, leading to even greater recruitment. HCFA director Bruce Vladeck (1995) has indicated that more frequent on-site monitoring will occur at HMOs that enroll many Medicare beneficiaries. In addition, greater effort will be made to educate enrollees concerning their appeal rights and the appeal process.

HCFA is working to develop measures of quality for the Medicare population and is collaborating with the newly organized Foundation for Accountabilty (FACCT). Not a creature of the health plans, FACCT is the brainchild of Dr. Paul Elwood, the father of managed competition, and some of the current major purchasers of managed care, representing 80 million covered lives. Both public purchasers, such as the Federal Employees Health Benefits Program, and private purchasers, such as the General Motors Corporation, are represented on the FACCT Board of Trustees. Other board members include representatives from major consumer groups such as the American Association of Retired Persons and the National Alliance for the Mentally Ill.

FACCT focuses on generating better information about the quality of health care by developing valid measures of the output of healthcare organizations, including consumer satisfaction, that can be disseminated to consumers throughout the United States. Founded in 1995, the following year this organization created five sets of quality measures focusing on breast cancer, diabetes, major depressive disorder, health risks, and health-plan satisfaction.

An alliance of purchasers, consumers, and health-policy experts focusing on accountability is promising. What they are attempting to measure is not related to the strong points of managed care but should shed light on the effectiveness of HMOs in handling difficult tasks. This kind of approach pays more attention to chronic illness than HEDIS or Consumer Assessment of Health Plans Study (CAHPS). The instrument is less burdensome to complete, and it is aimed at universal application so that the quality of care can be compared across all HMOs.

## QUALITY MANAGEMENT IN HMOs

Although these national efforts produce "report cards" on various HMOs, they are not designed to identify systemwide why problems exist and how they can be corrected. Independent of the quality assessment programs undertaken by NCQA is the movement toward continuous quality improvement, a spinoff of the work of the revered statistician W. E. Deming. This approach has been institutionalized in hospital management through the work of Berwick, Godfrey, and Roessner (1990).

Following these leads, the large HMO, United HealthCare, created a continuous quality improvement program called Quality Screening and Management. Using HEDIS-collected claims data, analysts identify problems in the making. Then medical record analysis provides the data to validate performance that can be improved. Management interventions are designed to deal with these problems. Finally, the same records are reviewed to determine whether improvements have taken place. This kind of work holds much promise for improvements in all kinds of complex health systems, not just HMOs. In fact, it is a technique of quality improvement found in many different industries, commercial businesses, and even government.

## LESSONS FROM MEDICAID'S MANDATORY MANAGED CARE PROGRAMS

When all Medicaid beneficiaries are required to receive their medical care from HMOs, beneficiaries have few options to go back to fee-for-service medicine. Several states that mandate managed care have recognized this problem and have attempted to head off consumer dissatisfaction by bringing Medicaid-eligible individuals into the planning process. In Oregon, for example, disability advocates felt they would not gain access to specialty care because of HMO rules and regulations. Consensus building was therefore a goal of the program planners in Oregon (United States General Accounting Office, 1996: 36).

> For more than a year before bringing disabled beneficiaries into managed care, Oregon's Medicaid staff held weekly meetings with health plan representatives, beneficiary representatives, and state social service agencies (from whom most disabled residents received case management services).

Discussions in Arizona as well as Oregon dealt with building common definitions of such terms as case management, medical necessity, habilitation, and disability. Arriving at acceptable definitions of these terms is very important to the disability community, especially when care that maintains functioning and prevents deterioration is denied because no improvements can be expected.

Three states with mandatory Medicaid managed care held ongoing meetings between the interested parties after conversion to capitation. Beyond achieving consensus, Medicaid officials worked with the medical directors of the various health plans to develop clinical practice guidelines and procedures for evaluating new treatments and technologies.

Aside from the benefits of case management or care coordination, the methods of quality assurance need to be able to look closely at the outcomes due to provider intervention, holding constant the various environmental influences that can produce better or worse results. Furthermore, to focus on provider intervention, better measures of risk need to be developed so that providers who have a disproportionately high-risk patient panel with a specific serious chronic illness will not be compared to their peers with a different case mix. Because risk adjustment is so difficult, HEDIS has not included it in its methodology.

When HMOs fail to develop a case management model or have no concept of interdisciplinary teams to deal with serious chronic illness and disability, then state departments of health need to make plans accountable. One way they can do that is to insist that approval of HMOs be contingent on contracts with specialty care centers, sometimes called centers of excellence, where access to services is not prejudiced by organizational cultures that value limiting expenditures over quality care. It is almost as if health plans have to be protected against their better features of rationing to keep them from denying access to specialty services for those who appropriately need them. Health plans have to learn about specialty care centers, why they are useful, and how to work cooperatively with them.

Finally, for measures of quality to be truly valid, plans need to possess "sensitivity to changes induced by conservation of resources" (Epstein, 1996: 227). Plans that use less may be placing their enrollees at risk while realizing savings in costs. Consumers need to be protected against decisions made to control providers because of the global budgeting produced by a prospective capitation payment system. When we are patients, we may not have sufficient knowledge or expertise to recognize the dangers of conservation, just as we often do not recognize the dangers of overtreatment in fee-for-service medicine and indemnity insurance.

## REFERENCES

Berwick, D. M., Godfrey, A. B., and Roessner, J. 1990. *Curing Health Care: New Strategies for Quality Improvement.* San Francisco: Jossey-Bass Publishers.

Department of Health Care Policy. 1996. "Consumer Assessment of Health Plans Survey. Chronic condition version." Cambridge, Mass.: Harvard Medical School. Unpublished.

Donabedian, A. 1988. "The quality of care: How can it be assessed?" *Journal of the American Medical Association* 250 (12): 1743–1748.

Epstein, A. 1995. "Performance reports on quality—Prototypes, problems and prospects." *New England Journal of Medicine* 333 (July 6): 57–61.

Epstein, A. 1996. "The role of quality measurement in a competitive marketplace." Pp. 207–234 in 3. II. Altman and U. E. Reinhardt, eds., *Strategic Choices for a Changing Health Care System*. Chicago: Health Care Administration Press.

Freudenheim, M. 1996. "The grading becomes stricter on H.M.O.s." *New York Times* (July 16): D1, D5.

Herbert, B. 1996. "In America: Mugged in the hospital." *New York Times* (August 8): A27.

Institute of Medicine. 1990. *Medicare: A Strategy for Quality Assurance*. Volumes I and II. Washington, D.C.: National Academy Press.

Ireys, H. T., Grason, H. A., and Guyer, B. 1996. "Assuring quality of care for children with special needs in managed care organizations: Roles for pediatricians." *Pediatrics* 98, 2: 178–185.

Kerr, E. A., Mittman, B. S., Hays, R. D., Leake, B., and Brook, R. H. 1996. "Quality assurance in capitated physician groups: Where is the emphasis?" *Journal of the American Medical Association* 276 (October 16): 1236–1239.

Leatherman, S., Peterson, E., Heinen, L., and Quam, L. 1991. "Quality screening and management using claims data in a managed care setting." *Quality Review Bulletin* 17, 11: 349–359.

Mauldon, J., Leibowitz, A, Buchanan, J. L., Danberg, C., and McGuigan, K. A. 1994. "Rationing or rationalizing children's medical care: Comparison of Medicaid HMO with fee-for-service care." *American Journal of Public Health* 84: 899–904.

National Committee on Quality Assurance (NCQA). 1996. "HEDIS 3.0 Draft." Washington, D.C.: NCQA. Unpublished.

Starfield, B. 1992. *Primary Care: Concept, Evaluation and Policy*. New York: Oxford University Press.

Stewart, A. L., and Ware, J. E., Jr. 1992. *Measuring Functioning and Well-Being: The Medical Outcomes Study Approach*. Durham, N. C.: Duke University Press.

United States General Accounting Office. 1996. *Medicaid Managed Care: Serving the Disabled Challenges State Programs*. Washington, D.C.: GAO/HEHS 96–136.

Vernon, S. W., Hughes, J. I., Heckel, V. M., and Jackson, G. L. 1992. "Quality of care for colorectal cancer in a fee-for-service and health maintenance organization practice." *Cancer* 69, 10: 2418–2425.

Vladeck, B. C. 1995. *Statement Before the Special Committee on Aging, U.S. Senate*. August 3. http://www.hcfa.gov/testimony/t080395.html

Yelin, E. H., Criswell, L. A., and Feigenbaum, P. G. 1996. "Health care utilization and outcomes among persons with rheumatoid arthritis in fee-for-service and prepaid group practice settings." *Journal of the American Medical Association* 276 (October 2): 1048–1053.

# 6
## Consumer Satisfaction

Patients' experience with managed care raise troubling warning signs
about the quality of care in the rapidly changing US health-care system.
—Karen Davis, Cathy Schoen,
and David R. Sandman,
*Bulletin of the New York Academy of Medicine* (1996)

Consumer satisfaction surveys have been conducted in the health-
care field for about a quarter of a century. Valid and reliable self-
administered questionnaires allow survey analysts to compare patient
evaluation of the services they receive. The instruments used for data
collection do not assume that consumers have enough medical expertise
to know when they are getting good medical care. Rather, they only
indicate that the context of service met their expectations. For example,
satisfaction surveys ask whether it was difficult to get an appointment
or how long past the appointment time the patient had to wait before
seeing the doctor. John Ware (1976) developed and validated scales to
measure patient satisfaction, and he and his associates have refined
them for the past two decades. By the middle of this decade, Ware and
his colleagues published results from a national survey of responses to
outpatient visits which showed wide variation in patient ratings by
type of practice setting (Rubin et al., 1993).

A more focused survey of prepaid group practice in the northwestern
United States was conducted recently by Donald K. Freeborn and Clyde
R. Pope (1994). With 375,000 members, the Kaiser-Permanente North-
west Region, a nonprofit community service program, has been serving
Portland, Oregon, and Vancouver, Washington, since 1945. The Center

for Health Research, an affiliate of this group practice, has conducted member surveys annually since 1975; these surveys are used to improve service delivery.

Surprisingly in this user-friendly environment, the problem of access, which commercial health plans identify most frequently, emerged as an important issue. The most striking finding in the monograph is that both physicians and members view access to routine care and continuity of care as the most serious consumer need (Freeborn and Pope, 1994: 126). And "both express frustration regarding various 'bureaucratic' aspects of managed care—such as the difficulty of getting through the system to talk with a physician and of getting a nonemergency appointment."

In late 1996, similar, yet more complex, projects were beginning to perform national data collection. With funding from the Agency for Health Care Policy Research, as mentioned in Chapter 5, the Consumer Assessment of Health Plans Study (CAHPS), a five-year project, was launched recently not only to develop and test survey instruments that will obtain assessments from consumers but also to provide reports back to consumers about these assessments. In addition, the project's final goal is to determine the extent to which these reports on consumer assessments are helpful when consumers are selecting health plans and services.

The CAHPS project builds on the efforts of John Ware and his colleagues and is moved by the consumer's abiding interest in the worth of differently financed and organized health plans. By 1980, the growth of HMOs was sufficient to command the attention of consumer advocate associations such as the Consumers Union. A May 1982 article in *Consumer Reports* (pp. 246–250) extolled the virtues of the nonprofit Kaiser Foundation Health Plan through the typical and predictable lead paragraphs of such articles about service systems. It described the excellent, intense, and successful treatment provided a woman with vaginal cancer. All her treatment was covered by her husband's employer through monthly fees paid to the Kaiser Foundation in advance of utilization of any medical services.

The same article summarized the results of two articles that reviewed the quality of care at HMOs versus fee-for-service medicine. Both articles, including one that was the result of a national study commissioned by the American Medical Association (AMA)—hardly a friend of capitated health plans—found that the care provided by the staffed-model HMOs was as good or better than that in traditional settings. The AMA study also cited the superiority of HMOs in providing 24-hour services, centralized medical records, ready access to specialists, superior screening of new physician hires, and an effective peer-review-driven system.

Even then, however, large HMOs were subject to the frequent complaint that they were simply "health factories" that delivered impersonal services. A 1980 Louis Harris and Associates survey found that "49 percent of fee-for-service patients say they knew their doctor or doctors very well, compared with only 30 percent of HMO members" (Consumer Reports, 1980: 250). Kaiser was already experimenting with more user-friendly services and researching comparison of consumer attitudes.

Overall satisfaction in the two comparison groups in the Harris survey were virtually the same, with a slightly greater percentage of HMO members (57%) saying they were very satisfied than the fee-for-service patients (53%) (Consumer Reports, 1980: 250). Little was heard in those days about lack of access to specialty care or denial of requests for sophisticated diagnostic tests (e.g., CAT scans) or treatments (e.g., bone marrow transplants), perhaps because there was less dependence on testing and fewer expensive technologies were available to treat life-threatening diseases. In addition, and perhaps most important, few for-profit HMOs were around at that time that sold stock in their corporations and printed their medical-loss ratios in the *Wall Street Journal*.

By 1992, with the public perception being that health care was in critical condition because of the financing and increasing inflation, *Consumer Reports* provided a more detailed and critical examination of HMOs, including ratings of the plan and consumer satisfaction data from more than 20,000 readers. Assessments by readers were in response to an overall satisfaction scale that was summarized in a satisfaction index for each plan where there were at least 150 responses. Additional ratings were made of HMO primary-care doctors, access and choice of medical specialists, and responsiveness of administrative personnel. Although the ratings of the plans varied widely, the overall ratings of both types of medical providers were extremely high for all respondents. Significantly less satisfaction was displayed toward the plan administration (Consumer Reports, 1992: 530–531).

Interestingly, the up-close and personal reporting found in the 1992 article, compared with the 1980 anecdote, was much more focused on the rule-bound or bureaucratic character of providers found in the world of managed care. All of the concerns now found in discussions of managed care, particularly gaining access to specialists, were raised in the more recent article. Only 3 percent of the readers complained about gaining access to specialists, while 14 percent were dissatisfied with the choice of specialist made available through the plan. Significantly, patients of primary-care providers who were paid on a fee basis were generally more satisfied with their specialists than those who received capitated payment.

In 1996, *Consumer Reports* was again evaluating HMOs in a two-part series entitled "How Good Is Your Health Plan?" This article was four times longer than the 1982 article and far more critical of the industry. Recognizing that a major transformation of health care had occurred since the perception of the "health-care crisis" of 1992, the authors raised the question of whether or not the health-care system was now not only leaner but also meaner. Again depending on readers who belonged to HMOs, their survey found that 10 percent of these members felt they did not get the medical treatment they needed. In comparison, only 2 percent of readers who had traditional health insurance made that response. A most interesting finding was that 18 percent of the HMO members went outside of their plan to get some medical care.

This last survey was also based on over 20,000 responses. The overall satisfaction rates were virtually the same as those reported in 1992. More problems were reported concerning not getting the care needed or being dissatisfied with the quality of care received. Respondents were most pleased with plans that either paid fees to primary-care providers or followed the older staff model that employed salaried physicians.

The questions asked are thoughtful, and the data collected from these reader surveys are handled well by the study directors. Yet the sampling techniques raise some questions. For one thing, the readers of this magazine are not representative of all people in managed care. Moreover, only those who wish to respond do take the time to do so, a process that raises questions about the bias introduced by using only the more interested as the source of information. In probability surveys of HMO members, the sample drawn permits all members to have an equal chance of being among those selected. Moreover, good surveys make an effort to go after those who initially refuse to participate, so that not just cooperative and amiable people become respondents. Some of these survey houses make an art of doing "refusal conversion," producing a higher completion rate or covering the frame of the sample.

In almost all surveys that compare HMO members with individuals who have old-fashioned health insurance coverage, the HMO members are less satisfied. In addition, consumers in preferred provider organizations (PPOs) also are more satisfied than HMO members, mainly because of the choice of physicians that their network provides (Consumer Reports, 1996: 42). PPOs do not use primary-care physicians as gatekeepers, which makes access to specialists a less serious problem for enrollees than for those in HMOs.

The rating of HMOs leaped beyond the tough pages of *Consumer Reports* in 1996 to other parts of the print media. In June of that year, *Newsweek* ran a cover story on "America's Best HMOs." The lesser known financial weekly, *Barron's*, also called for a "checkup" of the quality of care at HMOs. A year earlier *Bloomberg Personal* had set out to find the best HMOs in the country and found that few plans were willing (or able) to answer its questions.

The year 1995 also found the Commonwealth Fund, a national foundation in New York City oriented toward health policy, seeking to take the pulse of the nation with regard to managed care and fee-for-service medicine. In Boston, Los Angeles, and Miami, Louis Harris and Associates interviewed more than 3000 adults between the ages of 18 and 64. All respondents had employment-based health insurance and options in enrolling in either managed care or fee-for-service insurance.

Respondents in HMO were five times more likely to be dissatisfied with the choice and quality of doctors (25%), access to specialty and emergency care, and waiting time for appointments than those individuals with fee-for-service insurance (5%). Although most respondents were satisfied with their health plans, more managed care enrollees were likely to rate their plan as fair or poor (21%) than fee-for-service users (14%). This varied by city, with Boston HMOs getting much less criticism from members than those in Los Angeles or Miami.

HMOs did well in comparison to PPOs and fee-for-service in limiting out-of-pocket costs and the amount of paperwork. This is expected since HMO members do not have to meet deductibles before insurance coverage kicks in; and co-payments in HMOs are very modest compared to the standard 20 percent co-payment in indemnity plans. In addition, some standard preventative care and checkups were slightly more likely to have been received by HMOs members during the previous year than under fee-for-service insurance. These differences were not strong.

A major problem with HMO membership is the frequent turnover of doctors or the change of employment that ends a relationship with a regular source of care. Continuity of care is a problem, particularly if a person is being treated for a serious chronic illness. Access to care may mean seeing several different primary-care providers during the course of a year. This kind of discontinuity will less likely occur in mature markets where only two or three major HMOs have the entire market in a given region.

The Commonwealth Fund survey also found a surprisingly high turnover rate among enrollees, with 53 percent of managed care respondents having a membership duration of less than three years. This churning among members erases one of the advantages of managed care—the continuity that the plan can provide. Most of these changes were due to the employer changing plans or to employees changing jobs rather than to dissatisfaction with the health services provided (Davis, Schoen, and Sandman, 1996: 179).

One way to end up with more satisfied consumers is to educate them in ways to effectively choose a plan. Once they assess what they need, consumers will be in a better position to make wise choices. Medicaid conversions to managed care have led to the creation of a great deal of orientation materials for beneficiaries. Something can be learned from states such as Oregon and Massachusetts where state Medicaid agencies have developed booklets that not only list providers but also contain workshops to assist disabled beneficiaries to assess their health-care needs and match providers to those needs. In addition, the Bay State officials allowed specialists who were providing care for individuals with disabilities to become their primary-care providers. Apparently, managed care programs tailored to people with disabilities could serve not just as the acid test of a program's worth but also how to make accommodations rather than promote a "one size fits all" approach.

Another issue is whether Medicare managed care is good for elderly people. With an increasingly aging population, pressures have mounted to restrain Medicare spending. Following the 1996 presidential election, congressionally directed refinancing of this benefit will lead to more price-sensitive seniors joining HMOs. As with Medicaid and managed care, the state of Arizona has witnessed an enormous shift to HMOs by retirees. While only 10 percent of the 38 million Medicare recipients nationally are in HMOs, 33 percent of 613,000 Medicare recipients in Arizona are enrolled in these plans. The 1996 Gallup poll found that 92 percent of all Medicare recipients in Arizona's HMOs were satisfied with their participation in those health plans (Pear, 1996a).

Medicare-financed HMO members do not have to take out "Medigap" insurance to cover deductibles and co-payments for out-of-hospital care, known as Part B of Medicare. They can avoid filling out insurance forms, they have no deductibles, and they pay very modest co-payments upon visits to doctors. While choice of doctors is limited to participating providers, few complain when an expensive procedure is performed without hesitation or when discounted memberships in health clubs allow for increased exercising and improvements in functioning.

Arizona has also become the setting for a battle over consumer rights. Medicare managed care also may be the judicial arena in which the final word will be spoken on the rights of members who are not satisfied with an HMO's decision to deny them medically necessary services. As in other areas of health care, Medicare has been a standard-setter in the past. It may also become involved in preserving patient rights when consumers are unhappy about being underserved.

Traditionally, the Health Care Financing Administration has been the federal agency to which Medicare beneficiaries could appeal decisions by their health-care providers. In the past, the the courts argued that doctors receiving payments from Medicare were essentially agents of the federal government and beneficiaries were "entitled to 'due process of law,' including full notice of adverse decisions and a meaningful opportunity to challenge the denial of care" (Pear, 1996b; B15). Now a Federal District Court judge in Tucson has applied the same ruling to the rights of individuals covered by Medicare who receive their medical services in HMOs. Opposed by the Clinton administration, if upheld on appeal this ruling will encourage more elderly people to join HMOs since they will not be giving up their right to a hearing, add to the administrative costs of running an HMO to avoid appeals, and increasingly involve the federal government in such appeals.

In seeking a remedy for denial of medical services such as emergency care, home health care, skilled nursing care, and physical therapy, the specific services named in the 1993 class-action lawsuit brought by the Center for Medicare Advocacy, the petitioners were attempting to hold onto their rights. Now the government and the HMOs will be spending more time and energy in hearings and providing detailed notifications as to why a service request was denied. This kind of administrative cost involved in dealing with unsatisfied consumers will no doubt mean it will be more expensive for the Social Security Administration to contract with an HMO. The cost of running the Health Care Finance Administration will also increase, making health-care delivery more expensive in the future.

Sometimes patient satisfaction needs to be measured one patient at a time. This usually has nothing to do with the impersonality of the plan, the aloofness of the provider, or the quality of the specialists to whom one is referred. Rather, it involves the basic rationing philosophies of HMOs, particularly the for-profit variety. When run like any other business, an HMO seeks to buy the services and materials it needs at lowest cost, even locking in the price of a service by contract in advance of the need for the item. Under this kind of operating code— cost containment—an HMO deals with the rare and costly patient by getting the best deal possible. Never mind that the contract may call for treatment in a distant locale, completely disrupting family routines and creating new expenses for the family. Using the centralized planning mentality worthy of the former Union of Soviet Socialist Republics, one national HMO referred a child to an oncology center where she was diagnosed as having various blood disorders. Requiring a bone marrow transplant, this child from North Carolina was sent to Baltimore for treatment for leukemia. The local treatment center at the University of North Carolina was better qualified to perform the procedure than Johns Hopkins, but the physicians at North Carolina did not want to contest the HMO's decision because they were in the running for the next contract. As the child's oncologist and social worker wrote in the *New England Journal of Medicine* (Weston and Lauria, 1996: 543), the results were medically correct initially but devastating to the family.

> She underwent an allogeneic bone marrow transplantation which she tolerated relatively well, and returned to our care five to six months later. In the meantime, the older sibling was sent to live with relatives in another state, the mother was demoted, and the father lost his job. Several weeks ago, a bone marrow aspiration performed at our institution showed that the patient was having a relapse.

This story is meant to scare the reader. Clearly, the old adage, "A squeaky wheel gets oiled," holds true whether you are dealing with the motor vehicle bureau, General Motors, or your new HMO.

Patients with rare illnesses have been pioneers in HMOs, attempting to both ask for and get the services they need. As reporter Elizabeth Rosenthal writes (1996: A1):

> Patients with serious illnesses say that getting appropriate treatment within an H.M.O. has a frustrating hit-or-miss quality, depending on whether the H.M.O. happens to have arrangements with a doctor knowledgeable about the particular ailment.

Not only are the doctors affiliated with an HMO network not necessarily familiar with the disease, but they tend to follow the rules on procedures, even when better alternatives exist. Some conditions, especially in children, create enormous difficulties to perform even simple tasks. A child born with serious heart defects may not only require several operations but may also have very fragile veins, making drawing blood in a doctor's office, the standard way to do things at U.S. Healthcare practices, not the most pleasant way for a young patient. Refusal to approve use of a highly trained blood technician at a different location because it is an extra expense can be a serious irritant to the parents involved (Rosenthal, 1996).

Similarly, a child in need of prosthetic appliances may find the choice limited to a "one size fits all" policy at the orthopedic specialist under contract with the Oxford HMO (Rosenthal, 1996). Small wonder that people with disabilities worry about the care they will receive at an HMO. Will they be able to manage with the lifetime limits imposed on physical or occupational therapy? This uncertainty is added to the already existing uncertainties that people with disabilities experience: Will I be turned down for a date? Will I be rejected for a job? Will I be able to perform the job? As with the society at large, there is little room for accommodation at HMOs.

Patients also complain about HMOs that are unwilling to pay for innovative treatments, even when their own doctors provide them These proposed procedures are labeled experimental, and therefore, as with indemnity insurers, they are not covered by the enrollee's contract. Yet sticking to the tried and true does not make sense when the condition itself has not been treated before, especially when treatment can make a huge difference in the patient's quality of life. A cost containment policy keeps the price of contracts down, but it is not a big selling point when a plan is rated. Obviously, it is to the plan's advantage to get rid of the rare and costly patient where no clear treatment modality exists. Moreover, adverse publicity about these situations only scares away the population that needs extensive care over the long haul.

HMOs do well in the early detection of cancer, a result of ease of access and systematic screenings in annual checkups. But what happens when a person with a life-threatening disease in an HMO requires extensive and expensive care? There are some mixed conclusions as to whether HMOs establish restrictions on treatment in order to contain costs, consequently preventing members from getting the best care available. On the positive side, a Health Care Financing Agency study found that cervical cancer was detected at a much earlier stage in disease development among HMO members than in fee-for-service patients.

Despite this clear advantage, oncologists, especially those associated with cancer care centers, complain that members are not given access to these centers as part of their benefits packages. Some HMO members balk at the lack of choice of surgeons available and go outside the plan to find the best university-affiliated specialists. This decision may mean avoiding needless procedures because state-of-the-art remedies are available rather than getting treatment that was denied at the HMO. Again, the persistent patient who can persuade a health plan that a university-based cancer center will be able to provide better treatment can get the HMO to pay for it, using physicians and facilities outside of the plan. There is no way of knowing, however, whether the intervention that patients choose will have better outcomes in the form of extended lives. Sometimes there are quality of life benefits when some unneeded surgery such as a colostomy is avoided (Kolata, 1994: C11).

To some extent, HMOs are attempting to provide better care at lower cost by "carving out" certain kinds of diseases and turning over their treatment to organizations that specialize in only those diseases. In so doing, they are seeking to reduce the futility of primary-care providers' attempts to manage complex chronic diseases that exist over a long period of time. The Texas Heart Institute, for example, has been offer-

ing a packaged-priced plan for cardiovascular surgery to HMOs as well
as self-insured corporations, union trusts, and foreign governments
since 1984 (Hallman and Edmonds, 1995). Under this arrangement, all
services are bundled into a global payment package.

Such superspecialized treatment programs seem to be spreading. Beyond organ-specific integrated care programs, there are cancer care organizations that aim "to cut waste by applying rational practice
guidelines based on medical knowledge and a consensus of opinion from
a panel of independent oncologists. But there is a tradeoff for patients:
Their choice of doctors is limited, their access to some experimental
treatments is restricted and, in the case of bone-marrow transplants,
they may have to fly across the country to receive treatment" (Rundle,
1996: 38). Even in such "carve-out" programs, patients and physicians
at the HMO complain that they are restricted to the least expensive
chemotherapy, sometimes with noxious side effects.

Even with these innovations in treatment delivery, a major problem
for patients is to get information about their physicians and the terms
and conditions under which they practice medicine. This constitutes a
new hurdle in making an informed choice about which plan to choose.
Most of these rules relate to establishing economic incentives for physicians to contain costs. A physician, Norman G. Levinsky (1996: 533–
534), powerfully frames this new problem for consumers as it impacts
on the doctor–patient relationship:

> As managed-care organizations have grown over the past de-
> cade, the numerous barriers that such organizations can
> erect to the exercise of patients' rights have become increas-
> ingly important. Managed-care organizations introduce into
> the doctor–patient relationship third parties whose economic
> goal is to limit medical care in order to reduce costs. The most
> rapid growth has been in for-profit managed-care organiza-
> tions, which introduce business ethics into medical care.
> Business managers have a primary fiduciary responsibility
> to the stockholders. Both nonprofit and for-profit managed-
> care organizations must meet the demand of their largest
> clients, usually employers, for stable or reduced premiums.
> For-profit managed-care organizations must also meet the
> demands of their stockholders for a generous return on their
> investment and for growth in the value of the stock.

These factors influence the physician's decision making and also involve utilization reviews that are aimed at curbing expenditures, even
those prescribed by the attending physician. Consumers sometimes
find that cost-saving reviews by HMOs constitute more than reductions

of hospital days or the failure to get a referral to a physician. Sometimes the home nursing care that is offered as a substitute for in-hospital care can work—until it is cut back to what is regarded as medically unacceptable. Historian Jess Lemisch wrote an opinion piece in 1992 (A27) about what he and the doctor saw as a life-threatening decision, made when Metropolitan Life, against medical advice, reduced the allotted skilled visiting nursing care for his wife from 24 to 4 hours a day.

A more generic late-breaking problem that leaves many consumers unhappy is the HMO policy that encourages the switch of patients from widely prescribed but expensive drugs to lower-priced alternatives. HMOs make these decisions to save money. When a patient goes to get a refill at a pharmacist that accepts the prescription plan, he may learn that he is not getting Hytrin to treat his benign enlarged prostate but the less expensive Cardura, a drug not recommended for people with liver disorders.

Reporter Milt Freudenheim found that this problem was widespread and produced adverse affects.

> Patients and doctors describe problems in which drugs were substituted, or a plan refused to cover a prescribed drug, involving diabetes, high cholesterol, Lyme disease and schizophrenia. Over the past two years, medical journals have also reported problems when drugs were switched for migraine headaches, thyroid conditions, and epilepsy. (1996: D6)

Many such incidents cannot be avoided as long as costs remain the main concern of HMOs and other managed care providers. They will likely increase in number as HMOs start to care for more Medicare- and Medicaid-financed individuals, some of whom have complex medical problems. Some of these disputes will be settled only in the courts. Perhaps this kind of conflict can be avoided if plans start to work in partnership with consumers to shape the delivery systems under managed care and to involve patients in their own care (Stocker, 1995).

Consumer advocate Mark Braly takes another approach. He suggests that managed care has only made things worse for the health-care consumer, even though things were not so good before its proliferation.

> Managed care is a deal cut between those who buy (mainly large employers) and those who provide (now overwhelmingly some variation of HMO). Up to this point the bargaining has been mainly about what the big bill payers are most interested in: cost. Patients who have the most at stake don't even have the power of the typical customer, who

can take his business elsewhere if not satisfied. Their choices are so limited by the realities of the marketplace—by the inability to change plans at will; by the lack of fair patient appeal mechanisms; by the meager, hard to find, useable information upon which to base decisions; by inattentive, ineffectual advocates—that they face intolerable uncertainties about whether they will get good care, *even with insurance*. (1996: 1)

From his web site **Empower!**, Braly calls himself the managed care patient advocate. More significantly, he raises some good questions people can ask about an HMO before signing up, including: how many complaints has the HMO received and how were they handled? How many and what kind of complaints did state regulatory authorities receive and how were they resolved? How much of the HMOs revenues go into medical care as opposed to administration and profits? What practice guidelines determine the care you will get? What financial agreements and incentives are given to doctors in their contracts with HMOs? To what extent can a doctor be your advocate with your insurance company? Is there a point-of-service option available that provides conventional coverage (with deductibles and co-payments) if you decide you need to go outside the health plan's providers?

The doctor as advocate remains the strongest resource in the current health-care labyrinth. Mutual participation between doctors and patients can also help to avoid disputes when there is a clear understanding about the treatment alternatives available. To accomplish dispute resolution, patients need to know that doctors have retained their professional autonomy in medical decision making, something that even doctors are not confident about under the rules of managed care.

## REFERENCES

Braly, M. 1996. "Managed care: Who's the customer?" *Empower! The Managed Care Patient Advocate*. http://ww.comed.com/Hyp . . . r/articles/customer
Commonwealth Fund. 1995. "A survey of patients in managed care and fee-for-service settings—Three-city survey finds working Americans dissatisfied." New York: Commonwealth Fund. http://www.cmwf.org
Consumer Reports. 1982. "The HMO approach to health care: Are health maintenance organizations finally taking hold?" *Consumer Reports* (May): 246–250.
Consumer Reports. 1992. "Health care in crisis: Are HMOs the answer?" *Consumer Reports* (August): 519–532.
Consumer Reports. 1996. "How good is your health plan?" Part one. *Consumer Reports* (August): 28–42.
Davis, K., Schoen, C., and Sandman, D. R. 1996. "The culture of managed care:

Implications for patients." *Bulletin of the New York Academy of Medicine* (Summer): 173–183.

Freeborn, D. K., and Pope, C. R. 1994. *Promise and Performance in Managed Care: The Prepaid Group Practice Model*. Baltimore: Johns Hopkins University Press.

Freudenheim, M. 1996. "Not quite what the doctor ordered: Drug substitutions add to discord over managed care." *New York Times* (October 8): D1, 4.

Hallman, G. L., and Edmonds, C. 1995. "Integrated cardiac care." *Annals of Thoracic Surgery* 60 (November): 1486–1489.

Kolata, G. 1994. "Cancer care at H.M.O.'s: Do limits hurt?" *New York Times* (October 26): C11.

Lemisch, J. 1992. "Do they want my wife to die?" *New York Times* (April 15): A27.

Levinsky, N. G. 1996. "Social, institutional and economic barriers to the exercise of patients' rights." *New England Journal of Medicine* 334 (February 22): 532–534.

Pear, R. 1996a. "Elderly voices for Medicare repair: Arizonans find national lessons in their state's experiences." *New York Times* (October 29): A20.

Pear, R. 1996b. "Medicare patients in H.M.O.'s win a case." *New York Times* (October 31): B15.

Rosenthal, E. 1996. "Patients with rare illnesses fight new H.M.O.s to get treatment." *New York Times* (July 13): A1, B4.

Rubin, H. R., Gandek, B., Rogers, W. H., Kosinski, M., McHorney, C., and Ware, J. E. 1993. "Patients' ratings of outpatient visits in different practice settings." *Journal of the American Medical Association* 270, 7 (August 18): 835–840.

Rundle, R. L. 1996. "Salick pioneers selling cancer care to HMOs." *Wall Street Journal* (August 12): 38–39.

Stocker, M. 1995. "The ticket to better managed care." *New York Times* (October 28): 21.

United States General Accounting Office. 1996. *Medicaid Managed Care: Serving the Disabled Challenges State Programs*. Washington, D.C.: GAO/HEHS 96–136.

Ware, J. E. 1976. *Development and Validation of Scales to Measure Patient Satisfaction with Health Care Services*. Vol. 1 of a final report prepared for the National Center for Health Services Research. Washington, D.C.: Department of Health, Education, and Welfare.

Weston, B., and Lauria, M. 1996. "Patient advocacy in the 1990s." *New England Journal of Medicine* 334 (February 22): 543–544.

# 7
## Professional Autonomy and Managed Care

Today, doctors' everyday decisions are regularly scrutinized, monitored, and regulated, and their judgments about individual patients can be overturned by nameless employees of third-party payers.

J. P. Kassirer, Editor,
*New England Journal of Medicine* (1994)

Increasingly in modern society, necessary tasks are accomplished through the use of experts who give advice and expect their advice to be followed. Relationships with experts are based on the belief in the efficacy of the provider's technology. This technology is not a well-kept secret but is shared by those with similar backgrounds, constituting a professional community. Some professions become highly esteemed and are left to control their own members, determine relations with clients, and apply their skills without interference from those who might have a financial interest in the way things are done. The rise of professional labor is one of the longest running trends of the past 200 years (Larson, 1977: 14–15).

The professions remain objects of admiration today because of their moral independence and the perceived good they do for others and for society. To promote the social benefits or functional value of services rendered by the profession, societies in our times have encouraged professionals to form autonomous groups that are not beholden to a patron or the public and to set forth the direction of advancement of knowledge or its application. This independence does not mean that professionals do not face the usual pressure endured by those who perform other occupational roles. Professionals, a corporate group, have a triangular relationship to clients, society, and the profession itself.

Professionals, then, do not simply sell services, taking on all the other vendors in the marketplace in an open competition. Unquestionably, professions are highly organized occupations and have a monopoly over a given set of tasks. Their clients are in an ambiguous position because although they pay for services they do not have the special knowledge necessary to evaluate fully the quality of the service. The playwright George Bernard Shaw once quipped that a profession is a conspiracy against the laity, meaning that its clients are vulnerable despite the fact that they are buyers. In addition, faith and trust play a substantial part in working with someone who provides basically advisory services. Moreover, because of the nature of the problem—health, justice, safety—clients need to have confidence in the professionals in whose hands they literally place their lives and sometimes their fortunes.

In essence, professions have convinced the society at large, particularly elite groups, that they can help others to cope with the major uncertainties of living. A few professions—namely, law, medicine, and engineering—have gained control over their work environments and the requirements for entry into the profession. They have established techniques for categorizing the problematic aspects of daily life, and they have set up routine procedures for dealing with them. That experts have achieved this recognition or stature in our society may be partly a result of the knowledge base of the profession and partly a result of the justifications created to encourage people to attribute to them dominance over certain vital services (Freidson, 1970).

In his work on the transformation of American medicine, Paul Starr (1982) uses the elegant expression "a sovereign profession" to refer to a time when medicine had enormous autonomy, an epoch he regards as past. Sovereign professions enjoy a special relationship with society, create unique bonds among those with credentials, and dominate the terms and conditions of their work with clients.

For the past 30 years, physicians have enjoyed extraordinary freedom in a resource-rich environment to do anything they want on behalf of the patient. Upon reflection, these three decades were not only the Golden Age of American medicine but also what Bruce Vladeck, director of the federal Health Care Financing Administration, called the "gravy train years." An infusion of cash and credit made many things medically possible even if they might be medically unnecessary. An aging population, now equipped by 100 percent coverage for those over 65, made use of their Medicare benefits. An aging workforce, amply covered by health-benefit plans without deductibles or co-payments or even employee contributions to the premiums, were also heavy users of the system. While professional autonomy suggested that physicians need not do the unnecessary, there was little shared encouragement toward self-restraint. A self-regulating sovereign profession should be able to limit excessive service and heed the warning of economist Lester Thurow. Writing in 1984 (p. 1571), he said

> It will be far better if American doctors begin to build up a social ethic and behavioral practices that help them decide when medicine is bad medicine—not simply because it has absolutely no payoff or because it hurts the patient—but also because the costs are not justified by the marginal benefits.

Another reason why the profession of medicine engages in some self-correcting action are the labor market trends, given the march toward managed care. Recent labor studies predict an oversupply of specialists, an outcome that flies in the face of more demand that primary-care providers oversee a variety of patients (Jonas, Etzel, and Barzansky, 1993: 1063). The most striking trend is that over a recent 20-year period, the number of generalists dropped from 40 percent to less than one-third in 1991. Surveys of the medical school classes of 1992 indicate that less than 15 percent of the seniors selected a generalist career preference, with an additional 7 percent indicating certification plans for a general specialty (Kindig, Cultice, and Mullan, 1993: 1070). Interviews with medical students in 1995 suggest that many, if not most, will seek to become primary-care physicians, given the limited opportunities projected for professionals.

There is also an intriguing possibility that, with an expanded use of HMOs, the demand for *both* primary-care and specialty physicians will be reduced, especially if malpractice reform also takes place. Kindig and his associates (1993: 1072), though guarded in their willingness to extrapolate to the national supply, hint that HMOs may be able to deliver services with a ratio of three generalists to every specialist.

A surplus of physicians reduces the profession's capacity to remain sovereign. The oversight of medical work by payers, as well as presence of physicians who earn their livelihood as expert witnesses in malpractice litigation, was made possible by the oversupply of physicians found in the 1980s. The physician shortage of the 1970s which fueled the physician extender movement (e.g., physician assistants, nurse practitioners) and led to the increased class size of medical schools quickly gave way to the surplus of physicians found today, with a record 220 physicians for every 100,000 people in the population.

This surplus also helps to explain why physicians began signing up with preferred provider organizations and HMOs. Competition for patients became acute. Although the number of patient visits per person continued to climb into the late 1980s, the number of visits per doctor continued to decline. Access to the flow of patients became critical to doctors in the last decade since the government payers, Medicaid and Medicare, often refrained from raising their rates. Employers also sought less expensive alternative plans in the marketplace, seeking discounts from networks of providers. With cost containment the driving force in the reorganization of the health-care system, it consequently reduced the selling power of the medical profession.

Gold and her colleagues (1995: 1680) reported that, in 1994, 74 percent of independent practice association HMOs and 50 percent of the group-model or staff-model HMOs surveyed based annual remuneration to providers on the capacity of physicians to manage resources. The percentage might have been even higher if all the plans asked to participate had responded to this telephone survey. This kind of cost control means that avoiding expensive patients becomes a way of showing managers of HMOs good numbers at the end of the year. Moreover, doctors who have a patient panel of older and sicker patients may not be welcome into an HMO by other physicians and certainly not by management.

## PRIOR AUTHORIZATION

By the end of the 1980s, employers and private insurers were turning to cost management companies to review the performance of physicians submitting claims. They were looking to prevent unnecessary tests and procedures performed by physicians or charges that were out of line with what is usual and customary in that part of the country (Kramon, 1989). Certain frequently performed outpatient procedures, for example, colonoscopy, were subject to close scrutiny by these companies because there is wide variation among doctors as to the frequency with which these procedures are performed on virtually identical populations. Similarly, complex inpatient procedures such as cardiac bypass surgery, once unquestioned and considered necessary to save lives, were now reviewed carefully before being given the go-ahead.

Cost management companies employ nurses and doctors to determine whether a request to perform a major operation or an expensive test should be approved. Without prior approval, beneficiaries may not have their claims honored, or, alternatively, the insurance will cover a smaller portion of the bills. Following the lead of employers and indemnity insurers, Medicare in 1991 started a program to curb the costs of CABG through bundling the services in one package (Stout, 1991). This is one of the most common and expensive procedures that Medicare covers, with 135,000 elderly Americans undergoing heart bypass surgery in 1991. Reducing this $3 billion bill by 5 to 20 percent will produce real dollar savings for the Health Care Financing Administration.

Physician autonomy was challenged in another way. Insurers also took the lead at the beginning of this decade to insist that physicians prescribe generic drugs when writing prescriptions covered by drug plans (Freudenheim, 1990). Some HMOs even established a formulary that constitutes a list of approved drugs, based on both cost and therapeutic value. When a physician prescribed a drug not on the list, the patient would have to pay the entire price for the product.

Rising costs for claims have led some insurance companies to develop their own in-house review organizations. This adds to the administrative cost of providing health insurance, but in the budding days of managed care, companies like Prudential were pleased with the results. As we spy on what goes on in Prudential's Parsippany, New Jersey, redoubt, we can see how closely the company monitors and second-guesses the procedures selected by medical providers for 110,000 covered lives in the Garden State (Kramon, 1991).

> A typical day at Prudential's managed-care operation offered a glimpse of such an approach. In one case at the spacious new buildings housing the company's northern New Jersey division, a medical director concluded that a breast reduction was not medically necessary and that the patient would have to pay the whole bill.
>
> In another case, a Prudential nurse telephoned a doctor to suggest that he perform a gynecological operation at a surgery center in Prudential's medical network rather than the hospital proposed for it, where a smaller portion of the bill would be covered.

This prosaic peek at Prudential's inner workings only reflects what was becoming universal policy for employers in the early 1990s. Concern about overuse of hospitalization was at the forefront of this attack on the autonomy of physicians when it came to medical decision making. Self-policing did not take place, and the warning of economist Lester Thurow was prophetic. Sociologist Bradford Gray noted that "a 1987 survey of large employers showed that more than 60 percent were using preadmission review and about half were using concurrent review" (1991: 283).

## PHYSICIAN PROFILING

Starting in the 1980s, the situation for physicians was almost a reversal of fortune as far as autonomy was concerned. Up to that decade, according to *New England Journal of Medicine* editor Jerome P. Kassirer (1994: 634), doctors were empowered and few regulations impacted on their practices.

> Once upon a time doctors had nearly complete professional autonomy. If they completed their training, and were certified by a professional board, they were assured the respect and trust of the public, and virtually no one kept track of their professional performance. What a difference a few decades make!

Today, administrative and billing data collected by third-party payers and HMOs help to create physician-practice profiles, which is a more sophisticated way of overseeing the work of medical doctors. Measures of the process or care and outcomes make it possible to compare, let's say, Dr. Huxtable's work with his peers in the community or according to what are considered best clinical practices. Assessments of patterns of care could be used to certify physicians or to help them improve when they are doing too much on behalf of patients with the same diseases, or even too little! With refined data, a clinical performance profile can become a valuable tool in improving the profession's performance.

Welch, Miller, and Welch (1994) did an interesting analysis of inpatient practice patterns in Florida and Oregon. Utilizing Medicare's National Claims File, they profiled 12,720 attending physicians in Florida and 2589 in Oregon. They determined the total relative value of all physicians' services delivered during each patient's hospital stay. When controlling for disease and severity, Florida physicians used substantially more resources for each admission than did their counterparts in Oregon. This kind of approach could serve as a valid and reliable way of cost containment because it does not review each request for the performance of a procedure but attempts to feed back information to physicians so that their practice of medicine becomes more cost conscious without affecting their autonomy and concern for quality.

The profession and managed care organizations seem to be a long way from adopting profiles to retain professional autonomy while improving quality. Like the cost management companies that review individual cases, some companies are now in the business of producing profiles and monitoring performance. Little is known about the methodologies they developed for establishing their profiles. An HMO could be using these profiles solely to eliminate the physicians who make many referrals to specialists or order too many tests. Who is monitoring the monitors?

An alternative way of improving physician practice—the use of clinical practice guidelines—is little used, according to the survey conducted by Gold and her associates (1995: 1682). Guidelines are defined as "an explicit statement of what is known about the benefits, risks, and costs of particular courses of medical action to assist decisions about appropriate health care for specific clinical conditions." Moreover, to do more than pay lip-service to them, plans would have to establish formal, written practice guidelines and use them extensively, as well as monitor compliance. Finally, the plan would have to hold regular meetings to review with physicians the results of their use. Only one out of every four plans that responded to the survey systematically used carefully defined clinical-practice guidelines. Such efforts at quality improvement would be physician-derived and, by virtue of their nature, would have to be implemented by physicians. Consequently, some way would have to be found to compensate physicians for their time for performing this planwide function.

## FIGHTING BACK

Physicians started to fight back against the way cost management companies limited their autonomy. In 1991, most of this effort was directed toward state legislatures. Laws were passed requiring that these companies disclose publicly what criteria and procedures they use in making their determinations, that the reviewer be a physician, and that out-of-state companies not be used. All of these efforts make it more expensive for insurers to perform this kind of pre-authorization (Freudenheim, 1991). In no area of care has the use of what can be called "fourth parties" been more controversial than in the area of mental health.

## THE BATTLE OVER PSYCHIATRIC SERVICES

As a response to the increasing costs and utilization of psychiatric services of inpatient services, tight control has become part of all managed care plans. Concern was expressed in the 1980s that hospital beds were being overutilized for psychiatric patients. Psychiatric admissions for adolescents increased three and a half times between 1980 and 1984. The number of beds devoted to chemical dependency doubled during the early 1980s. The number of private psychiatric hospitals and the number of hospital beds devoted to this type of treatment also increased substantially.

With major corporations spending between 15 and 25 percent of their total health benefits on psychiatric and substance abuse treatment, it is not surprising that there is concern. Part of the problem stems from partial efforts to contain costs, thereby working, like a balloon being squeezed, to push demand in new directions. Another part of the problem comes from increased monetarization in this field. In health care, providers can create their own markets and surpluses by working around the regulatory controls. When Yale School of Management and Organization professor John Thompson developed the 470 Diagnostic Related Groups and introduced them to control Medicare expenditures for hospital stays, no effort was made to include mental illness in the length of stay averages created. Moreover, the prospective payment system was accompanied by another needed congressional correction in the payment system to eliminate lavish depreciation benefits as a tax advantage to the for-profit investors. The new accounting law reduced the profitability of community hospitals. Hence capital shifted from acute-care hospitals to private psychiatric facilities and free-standing high-technology diagnostic centers. Nonprofits established psychiatric beds to capture the well-insured patient, an increasingly scarce prize.

In no area of medicine have managed care components of insurance policies created more controversy than in the field of psychiatric hospitalization. Psychiatrists regard as irrational and adversarial the intervention of managed care companies in determining whether payment of long-term hospitalization will continue or be discontinued. They have also argued in their own journals that such interference is harmful for the patient's recovery.

> If the patient shows signs of improvement, the insurance reviewer may insist on discharge; if the patient is making no progress, the reviewer may still insist on discharge on the basis of the premise that the treatment is merely custodial. (Gabbard et al., 1991: 318–323)

Critics of managed care applications to psychiatric treatment offer anecdotal information which suggests that the reviewers were trained in Alice-in-Wonderland logic rather than in psychiatry. Naturally, psychiatrists have analyzed managed care from a psychodynamic perspective. What they have presented is a classic case of sociological ambivalence when they cannot follow through on a treatment plan that they believe is beneficial for a patient. In essence, they assessed the clinical impact of managed care review. If doctors take an oath to do no harm, then perhaps managed care companies, built around the use of medical expertise, need to be sworn in as well. Ever vigilant, managed care reviewers created uncertainty for the already vulnerable patient who was making progress—but seldom in a straight line. Following an analysis of the borderline personality, these clinicians suggest through detailed case material that there are serious consequences for patients who have difficulty processing this information. Moreover, treatment team members have difficulties working with a patient when they know that treatment time is limited. Families of patients are impacted upon as well when the reviewer gives a different view of the need for treatment. In sum, expectations of closing opportunities can create a sense of panic.

How widespread are these experiences? A recent survey by Schlesinger, Dorwart, and Epstein (1996) found that more than three-fourths of the psychiatrists who responded had experienced pressure from the insurance companies to discharge patients early. In addition, nearly two-thirds reported that hospitals limited lengths of stay, and half were discouraged from treating severely ill uninsured patients or Medicaid recipients.

Managed care in psychiatric treatment did not stem only from rising costs. There has always been some bias in medicine against psychiatry, but even medical doctors know that real diseases affect mental states and make people dangerous to themselves or others or create real suffering in people who cannot fully take care of themselves. Moreover, the families of people suffering from psychoses or schizophrenia deserve intervention and relief from their burden.

In this age of cost containment, insurance policies have become increasingly less generous in providing benefits related to caring for people with adjustment problems or mental illness. Even the self-insured giants like IBM have started to create limits for care in areas that are considered frills. But by no stretch of the imagination can mental illness care be considered a frill. However, some newer forms of treatment may represent excessive intervention once a diagnosis is made. There is evidence that hospitalization for the *early* stages of alcoholism when there are few associated medical problems may be unnecessary as well as expensive.

Despite this finding, there is still a need for basic routine care in the area of mental as well as physical disease. Insurance in general does not encourage early detection and intervention through benefits for seeing a regular source of primary care, and it is not so different when it comes to access to a psychiatrist, psychologist, or social worker. There is a need to demonstrate the *cost-offset* advantages of early intervention. Psychiatry and other mental health services are particularly vulnerable to managed care concepts. First, in the popular view many of the symptoms of psychiatric illness may be considered moral weakness and therefore not in need of treatment. Second, anyone who gets to play the sick role is *always* suspected of malingering in order to get them to give up the comfort and rewards of being treated as a person with unwanted problems. The person with psychiatric symptoms may be seen as doing just that. Third, even advocates of clinical care, such as Gabbard and associates (1991: 322), admit that there is a need for "definitive outcome studies on the cost effectiveness of extended hospital treatment."

In all fairness to the insurance companies and their reviewers, the focus of these refusals to authorize certain stays in hospital followed the development of private for-profit psychiatric hospitals, which were suspected of providing custodial rather than therapeutic care. In some states private psychiatric hospitals offered bounties for patients, violating the rights of ordinary citizens to due process in the course of an involuntary commitment. In other states, beds are filled in private hospitals with patients who receive no active treatment for alcoholism or drug abuse.

Despite these recent scandals and revelations that treatments for brain injury at special centers may be ineffective, some valid studies have been made demonstrating the importance of outpatient psychiatric treatment. Summarized in the April 16, 1992 issue of the *New England Journal of Medicine* by Leon Eisenberg, these studies show how depression can lead to more days lost from work than such chronic conditions as hypertension, diabetes, advanced coronary artery disease, angina pectoris, arthritis, back problems, lung problems, and gastrointestinal disorders. Depressed patients identified by a structured telephone diagnostic interview were worse off than medical patients in 17 of 24 pairwise comparisons. In a second study, based on a community-derived sample, the number of days bedridden for a sample of 3000 patients was 4.5 times greater among those with a major depression than in asymptomatic persons. And the risk of decline in performing daily activities by people with minor depression was 1.5 times that among the asymptomatic sample.

In sum, these studies show that disability days do occur for symptomatic people and that they need appropriate treatment. Not only is this humane, but it also makes good economic sense to do this since this treatment can lead to substantial cost offsets by reducing the use of other medical and surgical care. The medical community obviously has a stake in seeing generous financing of mental health services continue. However, real problems are involved in arbitrarily limiting benefits both in terms of the burdens imposed on families and the inevitable transfer of some patients to state facilities supported by Medicaid (Ruffenach, 1991: B1). Sometimes the hospitals and therapists have fought insurers at the level of the state insurance commissions, as when a patient who engages in suicidal behavior is scheduled for hospital discharge by the utilization review company employed by insurers (Goleman, 1991: D1).

Rethinking the role of psychiatry in the context of managed care remains a professional concern. The American Psychiatric Association has also published an anthology with 27 contributions, some of which provide guidelines for accommodation to insurers and fighting back against them. Of particular concern is the replacement of psychiatrists with nonmedical psychotherapists. One of the chapters calls for the training of psychiatrists to become the biopsychosocial specialists, but using their psychopharmacological acumen and legal right to prescribe to maintain their professional prominence, if not dominance (Lazarus, 1996).

Few providers or consumers would find serious mental illness a minor problem. Biopsychosocial care needs to be valued as a serious benefit, not a frill. How can this be done? Three basic principles can be employed to guide the construction of any managed care program. First, the managed care consulting company and the providers of direct care need to communicate frequently and to work in partnership rather than as adversaries. In some instances, reviewers and providers have been able to work cooperatively for the patient's best interest. In general, however, insurers do suspect psychiatric treatment, whether for inpatient or outpatient care, as being less valuable than care for physical illness. Some employers adopt this bias in order to save money on health insurance for employees and their families. Biased-based cost cutting may be counterproductive because counseling services for workers reduces days lost through sickness or absenteeism.

Second, the intervention should be proactive as well as deal with immediate distress. One thing that patients being treated for mental illness can learn is how to avoid stresses that trigger a serious collapse. It should not be assumed that the neglect of psychiatric illness means that sooner or later the problem will resolve itself. Untreated psychiatric illness does have its costs to society and significant others. And there is always the possibility that the intrapsychic stress will manifest itself in the form of physical illness or suicidal behavior. Unfortunately, psychiatric assessments and treatments are not viewed as preventive interventions.

Finally, psychiatric treatment can be accountable to insurance carriers. Utilization review is the form of peer accountability that has been generated by the American Psychiatric Association, assuring that necessary and appropriate care is delivered. The APA developed peer review services in the early 1970s to give insurers the option of providing psychiatric care limited only by medical necessity. This system has enabled insurers to achieve savings through cost avoidance in other areas of medical care. Psychiatrists review each case, working within guidelines established by the APA's *Manual of Psychiatric Peer Review*. The documentation of savings has been demonstrated with insurance carriers such as Aetna, Mutual of Omaha, and CHAMPUS, the federally funded program for dependents of American military personnel.

With these three principles in mind, an appropriate benefits package can be created which includes psychiatric care that allows healing time for serious cases and cuts down on the negative consequences of the failure to treat.

## ADAPTATION TO A NEW ENVIRONMENT AND A COMEBACK

Concern about the changes in physician payment systems has led some professional associations to try to determine their consequences before signing on with a health plan. National and state physician organizations have attempted to provide information for their members about how different payment systems work. In 1995 the American Academy of Pediatrics launched its Managed Care Resource Network, with 60 pediatricians from 27 chapters serving as advisors to their peers on issues related to physician compensation. Identified by state chapter leadership, these physicians are considered to possess expertise on issues, for example, related to transitioning in Medicaid managed care, managed care contracting, developing and working with pediatric single-specialty and multispecialty group practices, and working in a staff-model practice. These and other practical questions about the business end of practice have now become part of the professional associations' efforts to preserve the prestige, occupational autonomy, and incomes of their members in this new economic and organizational environment. As with other occupations and professions threatened by social and technologic change, the medical profession is attempting to adapt.

Clearly, the medical profession has lost some of its autonomy, particularly in the area of decision making on behalf of the patient. HMOs consistently do what they call "deselection," which is a way of politely kicking out doctors from their plans who are deemed lax in performing immunizations or other preventive interventions or excessive in using tests or referrals to subspecialists. Physicians need to heed the other early warning signs as well: inappropriate referrals to specialists; inappropriate emergency room referrals; inappropriate use of high-tech tests; and too many hospital readmissions (Clark, 1996).

The 1994 survey of managed care plans by the Physician Payment Review Commission, a creation of Congress, listed quality of care issues as the most frequently mentioned reason for plan-initiated physician turnover, with administrative or plan policy issues second, and utilization and cost patterns third. Clearly, health plans feel they know best how to judge physician quality and cooperation as well as efficient use of resources. Physicians can learn to live with this form of external discipline, try to survive in the shrinking fee-for-service market, or go out and start their own HMOs.

During the halcyon days of health-care reform, it appeared inevitable that professional autonomy would be lost to regulation. Few saw market forces moving as swiftly as they did. Many of the doctors in training at that time were resigned to working under these conditions (Rimer, 1993). Practicing physicians, who were more sensitive to the dynamics of employer benefits, saw their patients leave for physicians in PPOs. They, too, swallowed their pride and joined these networks and HMOs as well, taking cuts in their per hour earnings as a result (Belkin, 1993). Even physicians who joined HMOs were pleasantly surprised to find that, contrary to expectations, their earnings didn't dip and that they were still able to deliver quality care. But the one thing they expected to lose and did lose was their autonomy (Schulz et al., 1990). Delivering medical care according to rules was not what they learned during their residencies where they learned to take charge of the "case" for the patient's benefit. Moreover, going the extra mile for a patient in the form of advocating for a low percentage treatment that might be successful and prevent death may have no place in an HMO setting (Bossen, 1993).

By the middle of the 1990s, physicians were using their collective power to regain professional autonomy. Between 1984 and 1995 group practices grew enormously, particularly those involving 5 to 99 physicians, according to the American Medical Association's 1996 report. This growth spurt was particularly evident for multispecialty groups that could respond to the "needs" of managed care purchasers to treat a wide spectrum of medical problems and to the threats of these buyers to play off individual physicians against each other.

The financial environment has changed so greatly that on average nearly 20 percent of a medical group's patients are HMO members. Even more striking in terms of physicians' dependency on HMOs, each medical group has 4.6 managed care contracts. In addition, they report an average 21.8 percent preferred provider patients (PPO) and an average nine PPO contracts for each group (American Medical Association, 1996). The recent expansion of medical groups is also a result of HMOs avoiding both the use of salaried physicians and the construction of their own facilities. Marketing experts also have found that patients follow their primary-care and specialty physicians into HMOs. Consequently, health plans that recruit established doctors with large practices also sign up enrollees as well. Staffed HMOs that use salaried physicians cannot do volume recruiting of patients as the network or group model organizations can.

The growth of doctor-owned HMOs, as well integrated delivery systems, faces a difficult legal environment, which was originally established to prevent physicians from profiting by making referrals to facilities in which they held a stake. These kinds of fraud and abuse concerns generated state and federal legislation to prevent self-referral by physicians. Named after a California congressman (Pete Stark) the "Stark" laws basically "prohibit joint physician–hospital ownership of health care facilities and group practices and severely limit other joint venture possibilities" (Berenson, Hastings, and Kopit, 1996: 252).

If providers develop integrated delivery systems that essentially dominate a locality or a region, they may face additional legal hurdles. The Sherman Antitrust Act prohibits business arrangements that create monopolies and eliminate competition. However, the states may create enabling legislation to essentially limit competition in the name of the public good. Providers would not be allowed to conspire to fix prices.

Despite these barriers, physicians are moving toward emulating the HMO model. Many large medical groups can provide all the services found in HMOs and willingly take on the other characteristics of capitated medical systems, including assumption of financial risk. Some of the organizational practices that HMOs are accused of as being harmful to patients, such as financial incentives to primary-care physicians for keeping down costs through limiting hospital admissions, referrals to specialists, and reduced diagnostic testing, are found in these new doctor-owned plans. The AMA and state medical societies are helping multispecialty groups acquire the capital they need to organize either as HMOs or as care providers under direct contract with employers who send their employees exclusively to them (Freudenheim, 1995).

Given doctor ownership combined with HMO business practices, would access to specialists be any different if the HMO was owned by a large insurance company, a nonprofit such as Kaiser-Permanente, or even U.S. Healthcare? The same questions about hospital stays for psychiatric patients also come to mind when we think of financial risk-taking by physicians. In the 1980s, doctors in Florida who partly owned Magnetic Resonance Imaging diagnostic centers unhesitatingly referred their patients to such locations. Studies found that ownership led to overutilization of these facilities. Ownership may not reproduce the professional autonomy that by the medical profession experienced during its golden years.

The rules established by HMOs are intended to promote a "united front" to patients. Even disclosing what kinds of financial arrangements exist between HMOs and physicians is considered a proprietary secret and can lead to the dismissal of a doctor from a plan (Woolhandler and Himmelstein, 1995). A physician who cannot let a patient know if he gains a financial advantage by not referring to specialists loses a great deal of professional autonomy. Instead of doing what is best for the patient, no matter how sick, the doctor now faces the dilemma of being subject to a cross-pressure or role conflict previously not experienced. It is no wonder consumers and providers alike have appealed to state insurance commissions and state legislatures to remedy the situation.

## A POSTSCRIPT: HERE COMES UNIONIZATION

With the announcement in October 1996 that associations representing most of the nation's podiatrists were forming a union to bargain collectively with HMOs, the first sign was shown that doctors were not receiving the protections they desired from state legislatures and from Congress and would seek to protect their purchasing power and rights at work as those who work for wages and salaries have done in the past (Greenhouse, 1996). Podiatrists may be the new foot soldiers in the struggle to retain or gain back more control in the expanding world of managed care.

While the new National Guild for Health Care Providers of the Lower Extremities may not have the political clout of the American Medical Association, the AMA policy wonks are also looking into the feasibility of forming unions. Medicine is not the profession it once was, and physicians are angry about the changes wrought to their work, their status, and their incomes. All this has induced members of the medical profession to consider new ways of organizing, according to AMA general counsel Kirk Johnson.

> The fact is the union idea only works because of the frustration about the loss of autonomy and the interference by managed-care organizations. What doctors really want is some leverage, because managed-care organizations have taken control. (Greenhouse, 1996: B2)

## REFERENCES

American Medical Association. 1996. *Medical Groups in the US: A Survey of Practice Characteristics*. Chicago: American Medical Association.
Belkin, L. 1993. "Doctors fear changes may be for worse." *New York Times* (May 13): A1, B6.
Berenson, R. A., Hastings, D. A., and Kopit, W. G. 1996. "The legal framework for effective competition." Pp. 235–265 in S. H. Altman and U. E. Reinhardt, eds., *Strategic Choices for a Changing Health Care System*. Chicago: Health Administration Press.
Bossen, A. N. 1993. "We should call it profit care, not managed care." *New York Times* (February 20): F24.

Clark, G. 1996. "Heeding warning signs can head off termination." *AAP News* (August): 10–11.

Eisenberg, L. 1992. "Treating depression and anxiety in primary care: Closing the gap between knowledge and practice." *New England Journal of Medicine* 326 (April 16): 1080–1083.

Freidson, E. 1970. *The Profession of Medicine.* New York: Dodd, Mead.

Freudenheim, M. 1995. "Doctors on offensive, form H.M.O.'s." *New York Times* (March 7): D1, D7.

Freudenheim, M. 1991. "Doctors press states to curb reviews of procedures' costs." *New York Times* (February 13): A1, D3.

Freudenheim, M. 1990. "Insurers press use of cheaper drugs." *New York Times* (November 18): 1, 28.

Gabbard, G. O., Takahashi, T., Davidson, J., Bauman-Bork, M., and Ensroth, K. 1991. "A psychodynamic perspective on the clinical impact of insurance review." *American Journal of Psychiatry* 148, 3 (March): 318–323.

Gold, M. R., Hurley, R., Lake, T., Ensor, T., and Berenson, R. 1995. "A national survey of the arrangements managed-care plans make with physicians." *New England Journal of Medicine* 333 (December 21): 1678–1683.

Goleman, D. 1991. "Battle of insurers vs. therapists: Cost control pitted against proper care." *New York Times* (October 24): D1, D9.

Gray, B. H. 1991. *The Profit Motive and Patient Care: The Changing Accountability of Doctors and Hospitals.* A Twentieth Century Fund Report. Cambridge, Mass.: Harvard University Press.

Greenhouse, S. 1996. "Podiatrists to form nationwide union; A reply to H.M.O.s." *New York Times* (October 25): A1, B2.

Jonas, H. S., Etzel, S. I., and Barzansky, B. 1993. "Educational programs in the US medical schools." *Journal of the American Medical Association* 270: 1063.

Kassirer, J. P. 1994. "The use and abuse of practice profiles." *New England Journal of Medicine* 330 (March 9): 634–636.

Kindig, D. A., Cultice, J. M., and Mullan, F. (1993). "The elusive generalist physician: can we reach a 50% goal?" *Journal of the American Medical Association* 270: 1069–1073.

Kramon, G. 1991. "Insurers move into the front lines against rising health-care costs." *New York Times* (August 25): 1, 25.

Kramon, G. 1989. "Taking a scalpel to health costs." *New York Times* (January 8: Business Section), 1, 9.

Larson, M. S. 1977. *The Rise of Professionalism.* Berkeley: University of California Press.

Lazarus, A. *Controversies in Managed Mental Health Care.* 1996. Washington, D.C.: American Psychiatric Press.

Lewin, R., and Sharfstein, S. S. 1990. "Managed care and the discharge dilemma." *Psychiatry* 53 (May): 116–126.

Rimer, S. 1993. "Prospect of change keeps future doctors unsettled." *New York Times* (April 9): A1, A18.

Ruffenach, G. 1991. "Slashes in mental-health benefits start to hurt patients, medical officials say." *Wall Street Journal* (March 5): B1, B4.

Schlesinger, M., Dorwart, R. A., and Epstein, S. A. 1996. "Managed care constraints on psychiatrists' hospital practices: bargaining power and professional autonomy." *American Journal of Psychiatry*: 256–260.

Schulz, R., Scheckler, W. F., Girard, C., and Barker, K. 1990. "Physician adaptation to health maintenance organizations and implications for management." *HSR: Health Services Research* 25 (April): 44–64.

Starr, P. 1982. *The Social Transformation of American Medicine: The Rise of a Sovereign Profession and the Making of a Vast Industry*. New York: Basic Books.

Stout, H. 1991. "Medicine starts program to cut the cost of heart bypass surgery." *Wall Street Journal* (January 31): 23.

Thurow, L. 1984. "Sounding board: Learning to say no." *New England Journal of Medicine* 311 (December 13): 1569–1572.

Welch, H., Miller, M. E., and Welch, P. E. 1994. "Physician profiling: An analysis of inpatient practice patterns in Florida and Oregon." *New England Journal of Medicine* 330 (March 9): 607–612.

Woolhandler, S., and Himmelstein, D. U. 1995. "Extreme risk—The new corporate proposition for physicians." *New England Journal of Medicine* 333 (December 21): 1706–1708.

# 8
## *Protecting Consumers and Providers through Legislation*

Any suggestion that we don't support beneficiary protections or government regulation of the quality of care is just plain wrong.
> —Karen M. Ignagni, President,
> American Association of Health Plans
> (Pear, 1996b)

Their opposition speaks volumes about what is wrong with managed care
in America today.
> —Pete Stark, Member U.S. House of
> Representatives from California
> (Pear, 1996b)

When right-wing conservatives (and some moderates) say that some
problems are best solved at the state level, they are pointing to the fact
that members of state legislatures are very sensitive to pressures from
consumers, as well as doctors, and other small business elites. Not
needing a great deal of funding to run for state assemblies and senates,
these officeholders get elected by pressing the flesh of thousands of
voters and providing immediate responses to problems raised during
these encounters, along with phone calls and letters from constituents.

In turn, state laws designed to protect some interest group can make
a state hostile territory to a particular type of business. Nothing can
produce consternation in the hearts and minds of large corporations
with production capacity or sales rooms in many states than the efforts
of legislators to regulate their businesses. These regulatory statutes
make executives develop unique rules and operating procedures, stress
the need to acquire certain kinds of hires, and require other kinds of
activities that are not found in other states. Legislative liaisons from

the corporate world spend a great deal of their time in state capitals attempting to block change rather than encouraging it. State legislation can be geared to making things difficult for certain businesses, thereby discouraging them from entering the state or expanding their operations.

Therefore, much of the change introduced on the state level is in the form of protectionist legislation. There are also possibilities for creating new ways of doing things. Many of the New Deal programs of President Franklin D. Roosevelt, for example, were first introduced in New York State when Al Smith was governor. In dealing with crises, states also can introduce major efforts to implement certain health policies, for example, universal coverage, using the resources at their disposal. Efforts of this kind are watched closely by federal officials and the governors of other states to see if this "laboratory experiment" will really work.

This chapter discusses the extent to which states have moved through law to eliminate the causes of consumer and provider complaints regarding managed care. These regulations have begun to shape the discussion of the kind of health-care system we will have because lawgivers have attempted to reconnect providers and consumers directly, eliminating or restricting the interest of the HMO as the dominant and controlling player in the health-care game.

This spate of laws to protect consumers and providers has been brought on by the narrowness and rigidity of the HMOs. Since managed care is an attempt to reduce the cost of health care, it follows that disputes will arise between the plan managers and enrollees and, sometimes, participating physicians, concerning the plan's *obligations* to provide a rare and costly service, usually one that is not a decisive intervention that can extend life or improve functioning. As long as the technology is there, some patients will claim that they have a right to access it. Whether or not appropriate, likely to work or a great longshot, consumers will go for it, particularly when they believe it is covered by their plan.

In addition, the failure to identify the cause of a patient's distress may be due to poor diagnostic technique, and the availability of a better diagnostician might lead to earlier identification of the cause of the problem. David Ching sued his HMO when the doctors failed to discover the cause of his wife's abdominal cramps, despite examinations and tests. When Mr. Ching requested that an out-of-plan specialist be consulted, his health plan denied this request for three months. Following the examination by an outside gastroenterologist, it was determined that Mrs. Ching had colon cancer, but she died 15 months later (Rich, 1996).

The Ching lawsuit was based on the theory that the doctors' denial of authorization for an out-of-plan specialist was motivated by financial considerations since that group's compensation arrangements discouraged those kinds of consultations. The judge ruled that Ching had not proven that cost was the motive for denying the referral, but he did award him $700,000 after a jury determined the doctors did not take all steps necessary to detect the presence of cancer.

Managed care plans work under uniform rules that govern their providers as well as their patients. Since the providers in health care are the true consumers and generate the costs for what are sometimes considered unnecessary procedures and tests, providers who consent to work in an HMO agree to give up a large slice of their professional autonomy. In working under rules, the professional has become a bureaucrat, surrendering the independence that the professional as operator of a small business has. Moreover, as an operator of a small business that made out better when more services were rendered, the doctor worked under an incentive as perverse as the incentive to undertreat found in HMOs. It is difficult to determine which is more life threatening. Treating an illness that is not there can involve all kinds of powerful therapies with consequences that can harm the patient. This outcome can be prevented and should be even if there was a monetary reward to provide treatment. In contrast, allowing a patient to go untreated for, let us say, breast cancer is equally harmful, particularly when the consequences could have been prevented.

There are few better examples of the new restrictions imposed on physicians and patients than an incident in New Jersey where a team of anesthesiologists objected to their hospital's new contractual arrangements with an HMO. The HMO contract at Northwest Covenant Hospital called for the dismissal of the entire department if they objected to the terms and conditions of the contract between the HMO and the hospital. The physicians rejected the contract, and the hospital threatened their dismissal from the medical staff. Following a suit against the hospital by the 15 anesthesiologists, further threats of dismissal followed, and patient assignments for these doctors were taken out of the hands of the medical staff. In addition, a new group of anesthesiologists was hired, including a new chief-of-service (Nieves, 1996: B1).

The anesthesiologists at this New Jersey hospital see the administration's new policy as a threat to the quality of care provided patients. They have also experienced defections from their ranks, with only three of the original group of 15 now determined to go to court. The stalwarts who continued with the court action point to the loss of support as a result of the tight economic situation faced by physicians with "mortgages, families and commitments."

While anecdotes give us a flavor of what is happening, it is also useful to distill these incidents and present the basic sources of concern found throughout the states where managed care is creating a marketing revolution. The case against HMOs is made in the following criticisms from a consumer and provider perspective. The most egregious defects of managed care are not necessarily the ones that state legislatures respond to immediately but rather are those that are easy to get angry about because they make the HMO management appear cold and calculating, especially when it comes to comforting postpartum moms.

## THE CONSUMER PERSPECTIVE

HMOs seem to rattle enrollees when they fail to recognize the vulnerability of sick people or those who seek medical assistance. "Drive-through deliveries" refer to 24-hour hospital stays imposed on healthy and uncomplicated deliveries. Medical experts have long noted that infants pick up diseases while hospitalized in the nursery, and it's to their advantage to get out quickly. Despite the medical appropriateness of short hospital stays for mothers and their newborns, as of the middle of 1996, 110 bills were introduced in 36 states to extend hospital stays to 48 hours for normal delivery (*State Health Watch*, June 1996: 1). Seventeen of these bills were enacted by 1996. (When the presidential candidates debated in 1996, President Clinton, obviously having street crime and the drug trade on his mind, referred to these 24-hour hospital stays as "drive by" deliveries. Would that these acts could be banned by legislation!)

There is also the possibility that a federal law will be passed in 1997 that will allow women 48 hours in the hospital following delivery. This federal legislation is needed in order to regulate self-insured purchasers of health services who are exempt from state insurance laws. While introduced in Congress in the spring of 1996, this proposed law was part of Hillary Rodham Clinton's "Families First" speech at the National Democratic party convention on August 27, 1996.

Smoothing off the rough edges of managed care goes beyond limits on hospital stays for women who deliver babies. Patients who feel there is something seriously wrong with them want the benefit of expert consultation. Gatekeepers do not always agree with the patient's perceptions of their physical state. Lack of access to specialists refers primarily to resolving disputes between consumers and primary-care providers about whether a referral is required. Rhode Island and Virginia passed laws in 1994 and 1995, respectively, to ensure that an independent, external, and neutral medical reviewer be available to assess the appropriateness of a referral to a specialist. These reviews only deal with noncontroversial procedures. Michigan and North Carolina have somewhat different procedures, but both have established procedures without legislation, using the Health Department and the Department of Insurance, respectively (*State Health Watch*, March 1995: 2).

Again, doctors and patients may disagree as to whether they face a life-threatening condition. Denials of claims for emergency room use have been restricted in three states, and legislation is being considered in 17 other states. In order to contain costs, HMOs usually require prior authorization from a plan doctor, evidence that care was sought first at the plan's network of providers, or reviewed authorization following receipt of services. Maryland's definition of a medical emergency, for example, is built around what a "prudent layperson" would find threatening and dangerous. Such a situation would not require prior authorization for emergency room use. Similar legislation is being considered in Congress (*State Health Watch*, March 1996: 1, 8).

Demands for coverage or indemnification for care extend beyond the often-perceived unfriendly confines of the HMO. Insurance coverage if one goes outside the plan to nonplan physicians is part of a new law in New York State, one of the most sweeping protections for consumers enacted. This feature permits freedom of choice for consumers, particularly when there is a perceived need to continue to see a doctor who is not part of the HMO network. Known as a point-of-service product, it would allow consumers to get some reimbursement for consultations with physicians outside of their HMO, but with a deductible and co-payment cost to them (*State Health Watch*, January 1996: 3, 8). Under the new managed care law in the Empire State, plans must refer a member to a nonparticipating doctor at no extra cost when there is no participating physician with appropriate expertise.

This legislation has been pushed by a strong coalition of AIDS health groups, such as the Gay Men's Health Crisis, the Public Interest Research Group, and the New York State Medical Society. The problem with the law is that appeals of plan decisions are not taken up by any state agencies but remain within the HMO.

Consumer advocates have called for complete information about how a plan organizes itself, compensates providers, and permits disagreements to be subject to a hearing. Disclosure of the standards by which utilization and referrals are made, financial arrangements between providers and plans, and grievance procedures have been demanded by consumer groups as part of broad "patient protection acts." In 1996, only two bills made it into law (*State Health Watch*, June 1996: 8).

Applying to all managed care plans and not just HMOs, the New York State law calls for extensive disclosure requirements when requested by enrollees and potential members, including information about utilization review procedures, financial incentive mechanisms for medical staff, and the process for gaining access to special care and emergency care (*State Health Watch*, August 1996: 2, 7). The law also calls for additional information available on request, involving what prescription drugs are available and how decisions are made in paying for experimental treatments.

Consumers also complain about the bureaucratization of health plans and the various hurdles that have to be overcome before getting a routine visit for ongoing minor treatment or preventive care. Plans sometimes appear overly rigid in requiring a visit to a primary-care provider before making referrals for nonserious kinds of problems that only specialists can handle. Direct access to certain specialists has become part of state legislation in 56 bills with six passing, allowing enrollees to self-refer to network gynecologists and obstetricians, optometrists and opticians, dermatologists, and chiropractors (*State Health Watch*, June 1996: 8).

The state legislatures have not addressed a number of concerns of people with disabilities, including restrictions on access to appliances and prosthetic devices, lack of knowledgeable primary-care providers concerning disabilities in HMOs, and parent disappointment in lack of access to pediatric subspecialists. Most important, few protections have been established for consumers to gain access to specialists who have been treating a person with a disability but who is not a provider associated with the health plan in which he or she is enrolled.

Federal legislation is likely to be introduced in Congress in 1997, given candidate Bill Clinton's endorsement in 1996 of a bipartisan bill that would prevent HMOs from restricting discussions between physicians and their patients on treatment options and other medical issues (Pear, 1996a: A20).

While not taking legislative form in all but a handful of states, efforts to ban capitation and other financial incentives that create a climate for denying or delaying appropriate care are being pursued actively, sometimes by members of the health profession. California, which has been at the cutting-edge of managed care for several decades, has responded with two ballot initiatives which, HMO executives say, tears at the heart of their system of rationing. Two somewhat similar propositions on the 1996 ballot in California were pushed by the state nurses' association. Both would require public disclosure of the tax returns of health-care businesses. Proposition 214 would outlaw bonuses and other financial incentives for doctors to withhold treatment, prohibit HMOs from restricting what physicians can tell patients, and require full disclosure of all rules regarding criteria for the denial of care. Proposition 216 would establish taxes to make it more expensive and consequently more difficult to "downsize" the health-care industry or sell off nonprofit facilities to for-profit enterprises. In addition, new taxes were called for on "excessive" compensation from the distribution of stock to executives in the health industry (Pear, 1996c). Revenues generated from these taxes would be dedicated to regulating the health-care industry and to providing emergency care and immunizations in the state. Californians rejected both propositions by wide margins on November 5, 1996. Arguments against them were based on costs to state and local government for their health plans for civil servants and loss of tax revenues as the profits of health businesses would decline.

An Oregon ophthalmologist is gathering signatures for a voter initiative that would make capitation payment illegal in that state. Maryland, a state with a long regulatory tradition when it comes to health-care financing, now has a law that prohibits the practice of holding back part of a physician's annual compensation until the end of the year as an inducement to keep costs below certain levels. This incentive, known as "withholds," was banned recently in that state in health plans that pay a network of doctors on a fee-for-service basis but reserve final payments to see if expenses are within a targeted amount (Freudenheim, 1996: 1, 22).

Large employers have seen the rate of increase of the costs of their health benefits package slow down impressively in the last five years with the conversion to managed care. Some have opposed the initiatives and legislation in the states because they believe laws banning "withholds" or requiring full disclosures will make it more expensive to deliver services. The additional costs will then be passed on to employers in the form of higher premiums.

HMOs are also attempting to hold their expenses down by interpreting the Employee Retirement Income Security Act (ERISA) as exempting them from medical malpractice liability. The HMO trade association, AAHP, and lawyers for specific plans argue that HMOs have no liability because they are simply administering an employee benefit plan. Furthermore, where there is negligence the patient can sue the doctor or the hospital involved. The federal government disagrees and has filed friend-of-the-court briefs in several cases during the last three years.

The main legal issue seems to be whether an HMO's attempt to control costs by limiting care to what it considers medically necessary procedures and treatments can make the HMO accountable for an injury resulting from a failure to perform a diagnostic test or make a referral to a specialist. HMOs argue that they are not subject to state law because under the 1974 federal law that enabled employers to provide benefits without meeting state law regarding health insurance, as well as be self-insured, they are administering a benefits plan and are not medical providers. Yet HMOs advertise that they provide health care that meets consumer needs, not just the needs of employers, and that they are rated highly by those who use them. They also argue that physicians and other providers who are part of their independent practice association or who are part of group networks are independent contractors and not employees (Pear, 1996e).

Many of the laws established years ago are clearly incapable of either regulating the health-care industry or enabling new kinds of combinations and contracts that were unheard of 25 years ago when some of the last major federal legislation passed Congress. The introduction of the profit motive and corporate control in health care has produced new kinds of services and a new feeling of vulnerability for consumers and providers.

## THE PROVIDER PERSPECTIVE

In the early 1990s, physicians who saw their practice panels reduced sharply by HMO recruitment sought to join these provider networks. Often they were turned away because there were already sufficient doctors to provide services. Physicians felt they should be allowed to participate regardless of supply. State and county medical societies sought "any willing provider" protection through 69 bills in 29 states. Interestingly, a coalition of employers, consumer groups, and HMOs were able to block legislation in almost every state. Simply taking on all who want to participate was considered too costly a way to accommodate physicians who might not be appropriate for the delivery of managed care services (*State Health Watch*, June 1996: 7). In Arkansas Blue Cross and Prudential battled unsuccessfully against passage of the Patient Protection Act of 1995, which included the "any willing provider" provision. The law specifically forbids HMOs from excluding certain categories of providers, many of whom provide ancillary services. Thus, such occupations and professions as psychologists, speech pathologists, audiologists, and respiratory therapists, to name a few, are included. A second law added more occupations and exempted all self-insured companies organized under the federal Employee Retirement Income Security Act (ERISA). Finally, the Arkansas legislation preserved the "gatekeeping" system that is so central to all HMOs (*State Health Watch*, March 1995: 3–4). (This was mentioned earlier under direct-access protection to certain providers as a consumer protection.) Some specialty groups in many states have sought this protection because it preserves their economic viability if patients do not have to get referrals first from "gatekeepers." The inconvenience of having to see a primary-care provider, often only to get a referral to a podiatrist or dermatologist, is eliminated under this type of regulation of HMO policies by government intervention.

Some states, either through health department regulations or "essential community provider" legislation, have established the inclusion of public health or other programs in the kinds of services delivered through the HMO. Such regulations would require that HMOs contract with and pay for patients with special needs who are referred to existing programs at academic medical centers or university-based sites for assessments and treatment evaluations. These laws are aimed at preventing HMOs from substituting less expensive, less experienced, and less qualified providers for multidisciplinary programs simply because the managed care management is interested in cost control. Under the original Health Security Act and the various iterations that followed, such partnerships between HMOs and the so-called Centers of Excellence were required to preserve the quality of services available to plan enrollees.

Following the dismissal of Dr. David Himmelstein, an outspoken critic of HMO policies and practices, from U.S. Healthcare's Boston plan, a number of state lawmakers have considered forbidding "gag rules" clauses from being introduced in the contracts signed by physicians when they become part of HMO networks. "Gag rules" limit the physician's autonomy because they are perceived as forbidding them from discussing with patients therapeutic alternatives that are not covered by managed care plans. Representatives of the American Association of Health Plans (AHHP), a national trade association, argue that these rules only prevent doctors from saying disparaging things about the managed care plan and do not affect their discussions of treatment options. AAHP opposition to new bills at the state level has not been effective. Ranking second to maternity stay legislation, anti-gag rule legislation was considered in 1996 in 17 states and passed in 16, including Maryland, Colorado, Massachusetts, Virginia, and Washington (*State Health Watch*, June 1996: 8).

Related to eliminating "gag clauses" from contracts are efforts by physician associations to establish due process via peer review prior to termination of contract. Most HMOs dismiss or "deselect" physicians without any hearing where other physicians determine whether the provider delivers quality care at reasonable cost to the plan. Although the plan's medical director is likely to be involved in all these administrative decisions, that physician is an employee of the HMO and does not exercise independent judgment when it comes to personnel decisions (Clark, 1996: 10–11).

Consumer advocacy groups have also moved to buttress physician autonomy by passing anticapitation payment laws. The logic of this kind of restriction on how HMOs reward physicians is simple. Under capitation, physicians get to keep more of their projected remuneration if they use fewer diagnostic tests, admit fewer patients to hospitals, and have fewer specialty consultations for their patient panel. This economic arrangement is the reverse of a "kickback" situation where the provider gains something financially by virtue of shared ownership of laboratory, hospital, or specialty practice. If they were paid on a discounted fee-for-service basis, there would be less incentive to ration these expensive services, and patients would be better served because physician judgment would be based on the merits of the case alone. This kind of legislation will likely appear in some states in the near future.

The ratcheting down of expenditures on health care may go beyond elimination of waste. As rationing has its effect on controlling costs and hospitals become subject to contracts with managed care organizations that are based on deep discounts, reducing the per diem rate far below the usual and customary payments, there will be concern that hospitals may short-staff in order to avoid operating at a financial deficit. The concern here is that patient care is being neglected. There may be more interest in states taking over the accreditation of hospitals, removing this right from the Joint Commission on Accreditation of Health Care Organizations. We may see the emergence of quests to pass safe-staffing laws for hospitals. Professionals may lead this fight and gain greater esteem as a result of their efforts on behalf of consumers.

Bills introduced in the state legislatures may head off litigation when consumers sue an HMO for failure to provide the services promised in the contract signed between the plan and the beneficiary. Medical decision making based on "learning to say no" goes against the experience of consumers of health care for the past 35 years who have a strong aversion to rationing.

HMOs have taken on the serious and necessary task of balancing the patient's need for complex medical interventions and the society's need to preserve scarce resources. State law has so far attempted to deal with the most consumer-unfriendly aspects of managed care. The courts have traditionally provided an opportunity for patients who have been damaged through medical intervention to sue for malpractice and receive compensation for the pain and suffering undergone, as well as payment for medical bills incurred as a result of physician error.

The present concern is that under rationing the physician does not make a mistake by overlooking something that could be corrected or by performing a procedure badly but denying access to a vital medical intervention that might benefit the patient. No doubt, a "race to the bottom" could be going on, wherein the least costly provider in the HMO is held up as a professional for others to emulate. The courts will have a new set of medical issues to deal with and will perhaps have to recruit a whole new group of expert witnesses, physicians with knowledge of what happens when undertreatment prevails.

The courts may also have to consider whether state-based interest groups may be creating a regulatory climate that is so hostile to managed care that HMOs will decide not to set up shop in a particular state or pull out to cut their losses. The business climate could be ruined by rules that make it difficult for HMOs to use out-of-state utilization authorization companies, thereby requiring an HMO to create such an entity just for a single state. This would not be a very cost-effective move for an HMO.

Other matters that might discourage protectionism also need to be considered. A purchaser of services such as a large employer would not find a consumer-oriented climate hospitable. Employers might decide to leave the state rather than tolerate this kind of interference. Moreover, the "there ought to be a law" mentality only makes it possible for nonmanaged care providers to maintain their high prices in a marketplace where they are not competing with the HMOs. Finally, regulation that is there only for consumer convenience and does not in the long run demonstrate success in keeping people alive is not likely to help reduce health-care expenditures.

On the federal level, the Health Care Finance Administration (HCFA), the agency that administers Medicare and Medicaid and is responsible for 40 percent of all health-care expenditures in the United States, was seriously considering rules to prevent HMOs from using financial incentives to reward doctors who kept costs down when caring for Medicare and Medicaid patients. The HMOs argued against the rules, claiming they would have to rewrite tens of thousands of contracts and would put into practice the encouragement of unnecessary care. In response to these concerns, the government delayed activating these rules until January 1, 1997 (Pear, 1996b: A1, B6).

With rapidly increasing HMO enrollments of Medicaid-eligible and Medicare-covered patients, these rules would prohibit certain kinds of capitation combined with withhold arrangements and would require disclosure to the enrollees of these financial incentives for physicians. These rules could be a medically administrative nightmare for HMOs. HMO doctors might be working under several different kinds of reward systems when they saw private or government-financed patients.

This kind of struggle, one that pits the American Medical Association and various consumer advocacy groups on one side, and the American Association of Health Plans, the national lobby for the HMOs, on the other, continues on the state and federal level. The 1990 federal law under which these new HCFA rules were promulgated was passed at a time when the deficit was less of a concern than it is today and when HMOs were not seen as the way for both business and the national treasury to contain costs. The forceful congressman Pete Stark, the California Democrat who for years ran federal health policy in the

House of Representatives, until his party lost the majority in the House in 1994, attempted to proactively prevent the workable and popular Medicare program from becoming vulnerable to market forces. He feared that it would be less consumer oriented and protected if it was transformed into managed care. Therefore, he attempted to make it expensive for HMOs to move into this market.

Some of the state legislatures have followed this strategy of making it costly for HMOs to do business in their states. Providers and consumers also perceive that the capitation system, with withhold features, may produce a "disconnect" between the doctor and the patient. Through this substantial legislation, they are sending a message to the marketplace that both parties want to preserve the traditional ways of doing things as much as possible. The business end of HMOs is seen as keeping this from happening.

Apparently, the message is getting through to HMOs and their trade association. In the face of pending federal legislation, the AAHP in late 1996 accepted the idea that women who undergo mastectomies are entitled to a 24-hour hospital stay (Pear, 1996d). While arguing that physicians, not public sentiment, should set the standards for care, the president of AAHP, Karen M. Ignagni, has abandoned her loyalty to the Milliman and Robertson treatment guidelines (discussed in detail in Chapter 9), indicating that this is a fight that she cannot win. It is clear that the public believes that women and children deserve some special consideration, thereby making medical standards less important and acknowledging that biological functioning (birthing) and gender-related disease (breast cancer) engender certain health-care privileges.

### REFERENCES

Clark, G. 1996. "Heeding warning signs can head off termination." *American Academy of Pediatrics News* (August): 10–11.
Freudenheim, M. 1996. "H.M.O.'s cope with a backlash on cost cutting." *New York Times* (May 19): 1, 22.
Nieves, E. 1996. "Doctors take hospital fight to the street." *New York Times* (August 30): B1.
Pear, R. 1996a. "Clinton to name health-care panel, with eye on second term." *New York Times* (September 5): A20.
Pear, R. 1996b. "U.S. shelves plan to limit rewards to H.M.O. doctors: Industry wins reprieve." *New York Times* (July 8): A1, B6.
Pear, R. 1996c. "Stakes high as California debates ballot issues to rein in H.M.O.s." *New York Times* (October 3): A1, B9.
Pear, R. 1996d. "Managed care officials agree to mastectomy hospital stays." *New York Times* (November 15): A30.

Pear, R. 1996e. "H.M.O.'s using federal law to deflect malpractice suits." *New York Times* (November 17): 24.

Rich, S. 1996. "Managed care, once an elixir, goes under legislative knife: cost-cutting seen detrimental to patients." *Washington Post* (September 25): A1, A18.

*State Health Watch: The Newsletter of State Health Care Reform.* 1996. "New York's wide-ranging managed care law includes provisions that benefit chronically ill." *State Health Watch* (August): 2, 7.

*State Health Watch: The Newsletter of State Health Care Reform.* 1996. "More than 400 managed care bills, 110 maternity stay, flood legislatures." *State Health Watch* (June): 1, 8–9.

*State Health Watch: The Newsletter of State Health Care Reform.* 1996. "Rejection of ER claims by managed care plans prompts states to set ground rules for access." *State Health Watch* (March): 1–8.

*State Health Watch: The Newsletter of State Health Care Reform.* 1996. "Individuals in New York market now have Rx benefits, POS option in standard plans."*State Health Watch* (January): 3, 8.

*State Health Watch: The Newsletter of State Health Care Reform.* 1995. "Virginia patients or their providers can now appeal HMO decision to independent peer reviewer." *State Health Watch* (March): 2.

*State Health Watch: The Newsletter of State Health Care Reform.* 1995. "Arkansas legislature approves one of nation's broadest any willing provider laws." *State Health Watch* (March): 3–4.

# 9
## The Growing Business of HMOs

Some will contend that the market is already beginning to work—that health care costs are falling, medical students are entering primary fields, and integrated systems of care are being developed with private investment. Others will argue that the market has brought, more quickly than government ever would have, just those constraints that opponents predicted the Clinton plan would impose—rationing, limitation of choice, and neglect of threats to the quality of care—while still leaving millions of Americans without access to health care.

—John M. Eisenberg,
*New England Journal of Medicine* (1996)

How do HMOs become successful? The principle that operates in putting together providers and patients is to pass along deflation. Indeed, if inflation is passed on in a way where wages chase prices, then deflation is passed on in a race to see who can do it the cheapest. It is a race to the bottom—and that is precisely what worries both providers and patients. Can quality be maintained if resources are conserved?

As with any organization that creates some output or changes the environment in some way, the greater the integration of work facilities, the greater the productivity of each unit. HMOs are integrated organizations in the two ways that this concept is used in the literature on organizations. *Horizontal* integration means that providers with the same skills and interests join together to create a group of great capacity to see large volumes of patients. Administrative costs per unit of service decline when this form of organization takes place. Economies of scale enter into the picture, reducing the costs of such support services as payroll, human resources, and telephone systems, to name only a few important support services found in large organizations. More specific to health care, the group practice aspect of this form of integration allows expensive equipment to be shared among many providers, making technology such as a Magnetic Resonance Imaging machine less expensive to maintain when it is used more hours a day than when fewer physicians make use of it. In addition, a number of orthopedists can share ambulatory surgical units.

Where feasible, support staff can serve several providers at the same time, as when one receptionist answers the phone for 10 doctors, makes appointments, and orders lunch. Similarly, one office manager can supervise the clerical staff and also make sure that supplies are on hand for physicians. When services are truly high volume, a number of simple medical tasks (e.g., taking blood pressure) can be bundled and turned over to a nurse, a nurse practitioner, or a physician assistant, freeing physicians to do complex assessments. Sometimes primary-care physicians are replaced with nurse practitioners not only as the first point of contact but also for the treatment of minor illnesses.

With a large provider network, HMOs are better able to sell to benefits officers and other buyers of their services because they can demonstrate a wide variety of choice among providers who agree to accept their discounted fees. In addition, the purchasing power of providers increases when the needed resources are bought in extremely large amounts. Selling will discount more for the big buyer than for the small buyer.

*Vertical* integration refers to the extent to which the highly differentiated providers and units work closely together, but performing the functions each does best. Management seeks to avoid inefficiencies such as duplication of services and use of expensive providers when less expensive providers can be just as effective, and employs the kind of decision making that promotes the kind of care wherein patients get exactly what they need and no more. Hospitals and physicians are sometimes linked together through financial arrangements so that there is mutual interest in seeing each succeed. Matters of clinical care then becomes the more closely shared responsibilities of these two parties. To make these decisions work, a refined continuum of care can also be established, including ambulatory surgery, home health care, skilled nursing care, and hospice care. Coordination of care makes it possible to fit the patient to the needed service rather than provide a single service, which may be the only type of care available.

This modern form of integration is built on models created over 25 years ago. Pulling together a large number of physicians, hospitals, and other facilities was once the dream of health planners in the 1970s as a way of dealing with the uneven development of services. What this model suggested was that services should be distributed according to need. Thus, a given city, suburb, or metropolitan region might have far too many doctors and hospitals in proportion to its population, while some other locations might be underserved. Planning the distribution of primary-care services, small local district hospitals for secondary care, and large regional hospitals for tertiary care, for example, open heart surgery, as well as a university medical center for teaching and training, would create the right access for the entire population. Regionalization of this kind of care would mean that a network of services would be available for every 2 to 3 million people (Roemer, 1973).

Some of the nonprofit HMOs such as Kaiser-Permanente started to create organized delivery systems in the same decade as health planners called for more rational distribution of resources. When they began to provide health care for a large number of people in the same locality, it then became possible to create shared diagnostic and other services utilized by large numbers of providers. Having a great number of "covered lives" makes possible both adequate revenue sources and the need to plan services and promote articulation between units.

The logic of growth in contemporary HMOs starts with similar assumptions. The first step in being a successful HMO today is to get a contract with employers who can deliver a large number of lives to cover. This requires being willing to offer deep discounts to attract customers. Benefits officers are usually seeking to beat the national average expenditures for both HMO coverage and traditional indemnity insurance coverage. Because there is a great deal of competition among the HMOs today in metropolitan areas, the corporations are finding it is a buyer's market.

Still, these plans have to be attractive to employees and their families. Since employers often offer employees a menu of several options, HMOs need an assist from the employer to get employees to sign up. This assist usually comes from lower out-of-pocket costs for each family, both from lower deductions than indemnity coverage from the weekly or monthly paycheck and lower co-payments and no deductibles. These can be powerful incentives in a time when wages and salaries are stagnant. Saving money is another way of increasing a family's purchasing power. Some corporations will encourage their employees to enroll in the lowest cost HMO by picking up a greater percentage of the total charges by the health plan than in the more expensive alternatives.

Despite these incentives, some families are still reluctant to leave indemnity insurance that covers an esteemed provider. Patients with serious medical problems or young children will often be loyal to their physicians. HMOs also learned throughout the 1990s that potential enrollees are discouraged when their own primary-care doctor or specialist is not listed in an HMO's stable of providers. To encourage recruitment, HMOs often attempt to bring into their network the local doctors near a company that can give them many enrollees. It is of particular use to sign up a large number of pediatricians known to the employees. Maintaining those relationships is important to parents. If those familiar and well-known providers are on the HMO's list, then the decision to join up becomes an easy one. When an enrollee has access to the same doctor at less cost, how can one refuse to enroll?

There is yet another inducement for joining an HMO. A point-of-service option assures the enrollees that any doctor who accepts indemnity insurance will be available to them if they cannot find what they want within the network. Of course, they must pay some substantial first-dollar or deductible costs and usually also a 20 percent co-payment for every visit until some large amount of out-of-pocket expenses have been incurred.

This kind of option—a safety feature for those who are concerned about being locked in to a panel of doctors—is not used that much, but it is reassuring to know that some insurance coverage is available if some recondite problem cannot be managed within the HMO's arsenal of providers. It can also be said that the "point-of-service" feature helps to convert members into believers. This backup indemnity insurance provides a bridge back to trusted providers who may not join the network. If an HMO enrollee is in the middle of treatment with a non-network provider, that treatment can continue while the rest of the family takes advantage of the care available within the network. This feature is a way of creating confidence in a new and untried system of health-care delivery.

Similarly, the employer who signs on with one HMO may not be guaranteed the same price for a new contract in the future. Usually, when a decision must be made, a quick study is made of the indemnity insurance selling price and a rapid calculation is determined as to how much to charge the employers. The price that is quoted will usually be lower than the price quoted for indemnity insurance, but it will be close to that quote. The business pages of the daily newspaper sometimes refer to this as "shadow pricing." Sometimes rates are cut dramatically when a large number of subscribers signs on in one fell swoop.

Different sales techniques can be used to recruit senior citizens who are eligible for Medicare and who must be signed on one at a time. Like banks that give away toaster ovens and luggage, HMOs have taken the gift route to bring in this sector of the population. Recruiting the elderly population has a substantial financial incentive for HMOs since they are paid at a rate that is 95 percent of the average expenses incurred by the total Medicare-covered population. Since the mean average includes the costs to the Health Care Financing Administration of many very sick individuals who receive a disproportionate share of all the dollars spent on the Medicare population, the typical senior enrollee in an HMO incurs costs well below that figure (Kilborn, 1996).

The HMO movement has been helped along by the use of capital accumulated by the large American health insurance corporations. Cigna of Connecticut was once a straight indemnity insurance company but rapidly reorganized itself into one of the largest vendors of managed care plans. Financial analyst and reporter Peter Kerr observes that this company is organizing a medical network that will dominate health care in the twenty-first century.

> Since 1984, Cigna has organized about 150 networks that together serve more than 2.6 million people nationwide. The company will not say how much it has invested in managed care. But after years of losses its managed-care operations are now profitable and health plans are responsible for the lion's share of the company's earnings. (Kerr, 1993, Section 3:6)

Increasingly, HMOs and other managed care plans like Cigna, by driving out or buying out weaker competition, have created mature markets in metropolitan areas, wherein five or six very large plans hold most of the market share. Plans may acquire hospitals, medical practices, and other elements of a delivery system in an area where they do a great deal of business. In some parts of the United States, consumers and providers have widely accepted the HMO model. Gains in integrating services, as well as changing styles of medical practice, were noted in California at the beginning of the decade. The result has been less use of diagnostic testing and referral to specialists (Freudenheim, 1991).

Sometimes this kind of alignment becomes a liability. In Minneapolis, the home of some of the largest HMOs in the country, employers started to take another look at the HMOs with which they had contracts and to seek quality, not just savings. These giant corporations are starting to negotiate directly with medical groups and hospitals in the metropolitan area of the Twin Cities to promote new approaches to care (Winslow, 1995). One such provider network, Health Systems Minnesota, posted a doctor full time on a rotating basis at its participating hospital. Data on over 400 patients showed that the presence of this physician in the wards shortened hospital stays and substantially reduced specialty consultations, thereby cutting overall costs per admission by 20 percent. Patients were pleased with the care they received, even though they did not get treated and monitored by their own doctors.

The battle for market share can also mean that HMO profits may be limited as charges to employers are kept low. With earnings down, companies whose stock is traded publicly may find that the price of their shares in the stock market will decline. Other factors have to do with unpredicted changes in physician-practice styles related to prescribing or to hospitalizing patients, therein creating greater costs for the for-profits than were anticipated when they offered a proposal to corporations to become one of their health plans (Freudenheim, 1996).

## LEARNING TO SAY NO

In the past, doctors were encouraged to do more for the patient for financial reasons and, to some extent, for fear of losing patients who perceived that their complaints required attention. The incentives are reversed today in HMOs and managed care plans, and providers need to convince patients that less is more. What this means is that they need to justify their medical decisions to skeptical patients who often feel they are being ignored because HMOs do better as an enterprise when they are cost conscious.

Again in California, we find a living laboratory concerning how managed care is transforming the delivery of services. James C. Robinson (1996) measured the impact of HMOs on hospital capacity and utilization between 1983 and 1993. Using multivariate analysis, he studied private nonprofit and for-profit hospitals in the Golden State with 25 or more beds. He found that HMO market penetration accelerated the substitution of outpatient for inpatient surgery and the shift from acute to subacute inpatient days and reduced psychiatric hospitalization.

Managed care has pushed the acute-care hospital from the core to the periphery of the delivery system. This change did not happen without guidance from experts on health outcomes. Not surprisingly, some companies create standards for clinical practice, telling doctors what to treat and how much treatment to provide. In addition, corporations such as the 48-year-old firm Milliman and Robertson consult with the for-profit and nonprofit HMOs to advise them on what to cover and what not to cover. Needless to say, many doctors treat these guidelines as irrelevant to good medical practice since they regard each patient as unique. The American Medical Association, which has not produced its own guidelines, has fought the Milliman guidelines as unnecessary. Still, the AMA appears to be covering all bases: There is a report that the AMA is interested in buying the company as a way to set standards under its aegis.

The standards are set through extensive reviews of the medical literature and the study of medical records or charts to determine what works and what does not. The Milliman guidelines cover hospital admission and stays, office treatments, home health care, and recovery times for individuals before returning to work. Additional volumes in the future will address medication issues and dental treatments.

Run by the iconoclastic Dr. Richard L. Doyle, Milliman and Robertson depend on nine doctors and nine nurses to create guidelines. The focus of much of their work is on reducing what they considered unnecessary hospital days. Since hospital per diem costs averaged $1500 by the mid-1990s, the savings to health plans by reducing stays can be quite substantial. Throughout the country, use of these guidelines has reduced the number of days patients stay by one-third, particularly in California and the Middle West. The East Coast physician groups have resisted the use of length-of-stay guidelines and have sought to introduce legal challenges to their application in medical decision making (Myerson, 1995).

The use of clinical treatment guidelines is only one way that HMOs keep doctors from providing care that may get to be expensive and, at least according to these standards, not very effective. HMOs also attempt to manage physician behavior by recruiting and selecting only those physicians who can work under these kinds of restrictions. Any health delivery structure—or conditions that create uniform patterns of behavior—requires selection and training so that management can get physicians who can work under rules. This means that younger, rather than older, physicians will be recruited since they are less set in their ways. A strong reliance on primary-care physicians, particularly those with training in family practice medicine, means that they will employ providers who are less prone to test, hospitalize, and refer to specialists.

A 1994 national telephone survey of 108 managed care plans described the different kinds of arrangements made with physicians according to the type of provider organization established (Gold et al., 1995). Recruitment standards vary, with the group or staff models having more demanding requirements than are found in independent practice associations (IPAs) or preferred provider organizations (PPOs). Once accepted, turnover rates are low in all models of organizing physicians.

According to the Gold study, most HMOs require primary-care providers and specialists to go through a certification procedure. This procedure can "deselect" or weed out those with histories that predict they won't be cooperative or those who have been dropped from the practitioner roles of other health plans. Then, physicians need to learn how to work under new financial incentives.

> Among the network or IPA HMOs, 84 percent had some sharing of risk with primary care physicians; 56 percent used

capitation as a primary method of payment; and 28 percent used fee-for-service payments in some form along with withholding or bonuses. (p. 1680)

IPAs were most likely to use consumer satisfaction information to determine bonus payments, while group and staff HMOs rewarded productivity and tenure. Practice and utilization management were generally guided by policy, peer review, and outcome studies.

More than 95 percent of the HMOs and 62 percent of the PPOs had a written quality-assurance plan, a quality-assurance committee, and a patient-grievance system. Seventy-nine percent of the group or staff HMOs and 70 percent of the network or IPA HMOs required outcome studies for particular clinical conditions, had targeted quality improvement initiatives, and used outcome studies to identify needs for improvement and to gauge success. (p. 1681)

The most recent form of organizing physicians is through independent and integrated medical groups. Clearly, this type of arrangement allows physicians to establish greater bargaining power with HMOs. In this way, doctors have attempted to resist the market pressures of HMOs by organizing into their own networks as well as seeking legislation to protect their rights or to limit financial incentives that encourage cost containment. Large medical groups in California have contracted with HMOs through capitation to provide integrated medical services on a per-member per-month basis. Each group is financially at risk for the costs of care. As Robinson and Casalino report, "These groups manage the full spectrum of care, including the services provided by their own physicians and those provided by outside physicians, hospitals, and ancillary organizations" (1995: 1684). These medical groups compensate physicians through a fixed salary, with bonuses determined by physician productivity, patient satisfaction, and group profitability. Because these groups own their own hospitals, they can receive HMO payments for hospital as well as professional services.

These groups were successful in keeping the rate of hospitalization and patient visits well below the national average for HMO patients as well for non-HMO patients. Most important, Robinson and Casalino were able to show that management techniques made a difference in cost containment.

Medical directors and physician committees at these California groups performed their own reviews of utilization and its management rather than hire consultation firms to perform these tasks. Using clinical information, this approach is cooperative rather than adversarial.

Most important, it takes management functions out of the hands of the HMOs and allows doctors to review and reward doctors. This arrangement eliminates the individualized negotiations that go on between HMOs and physicians in most state plans.

When doctors got together in the past to agree on what price to charge, the Federal Trade Commission often saw this practice as price-fixing, which is a clear violation of federal antitrust law. New rulings from the Commission suggest that when it is deemed to be in the public or consumer interest for these combinations occur, such arrangements will be considered legal (Pear, 1996). These physician networks are viewed as encouraging competition, as when doctors combine to sell their services directly to an employer, thereby eliminating HMOs as the broker.

Under antitrust law, physicians could create a provider network only if they also assumed financial risk. Under the new rulings of the Justice Department, doctors could be paid on a fee-for-service basis, and benefit for consumers would take place in the form of better services through competition. By pooling information on prices and costs, provider networks would be in a better position to determine price setting.

HMOs not only contract with existing integrated medical systems but also contract on a capitation basis with highly specialized provider systems that concentrate on delivery of services to people with specific diseases or behavioral problems. Under a "carve-out" arrangement, these contractors agree to assume all financial risk for the care of a particular population whose care the provider network or a staffed HMO considers to be very expensive. A capitation charge for the entire panel of "covered lives" generates the payment to the specialized provider program. From the HMO's perspective, this shedding of tasks allows management to lock in their costs for the coming year, making expenditures more predictable. This enables them to offer contracts that will be less likely to lose money through miscalculation of costs.

An HMO may contract with a company to provide all mental health services, ranging from psychiatric hospitalization, outpatient therapy, and even testing of children suspected of having developmental lags. All management and delivery of these services are in the hands of the specialized provider. Some of these mental health service programs are considered controversial because of the limits imposed on hospital days for psychiatric patients, considered to need more time to recover, or because family may regard them as dangerous to themselves or others.

More recently, HMOs have contracted with a real upstart in the cancer treatment field, a company run by Dr. Bernard Salick. This physician is applying the principles he learned in running dialysis units and his experience in getting care for his daughter who had bone cancer as a six year old. Starting on the West Coast, where many innovations in the United States have emerged, Salick has moved into large-volume cancer markets in Florida and New York City. His seven-day-a-week, 24-hour-a-day treatment services make maximum use of facilities, thereby driving down the cost of service delivery to each patient. Because his operation has high volume, he can also get deep discounts from pharmaceutical manufacturers and other suppliers (Rosenthal, 1996).

As you might have guessed, not everyone is happy with this innovative program. Some cities with well-established programs that provide services and train oncologists are deeply threatened by the loss of revenues once the HMOs turn to Salick Health Care to care for those with catastrophic illness. Moreover, Salick has lured away some top specialists to direct these centers attached to prominent hospitals that had little treatment capacity in this area before his arrival. Further, hospices will also lose referrals because Salick also offers palliative care as part of a comprehensive package to HMOs.

Analysts of the new forms of HMOs suggest that the real advances in managed care management come from responding to the two major components of the system: the providers and the consumers. Like any complex organization, there are internal and external markets that must be satisfied and controlled at the same time.

Providers need to learn how to work within a system that downplays heroic intervention, an attribute that physicians acquire during medical education and training. They need to make good decisions, based on the limited resources they have available and the knowledge of what works and what is ineffective. This information must be kept continuously fresh in order to achieve the best outcomes. If the age of big government is over, so is the age of overtreatment and lack of concern for cost. Plans may need to do some medical "unlearning" as well as training about the rules and regulations of being a participating provider.

Good providers also need information on how well they are doing compared to their peers. It is critical that information be available in order to maintain the goals and objectives of the commercial HMO—quality care at reasonable cost, with a profit. The nonprofits also need to learn how to use information effectively to improve care coordination and to determine whether the desired results are occurring.

Information is also useful in determining the price of the health plan the HMO will sell in the marketplace. Consumers will be more receptive when they are given some choice of plans, perhaps available at the same seller. Plans should not consider "one size fits all," since the American consumer looks for choice, even when the distinctions between products may be minimal.

The business practices of HMOs and their collaborators helped reduce the rise of health-care costs in the 1990s during President Clinton's first term in office. Physician income declined in 1994, with specialists taking a 5 percent reduction. The HMOs clearly have had the upper hand in bargaining, and even those physicians who do not participate in managed care plans have had to keep their fees down to avoid losing patients to HMOs.

Yet the market forces that shape our health-care system have not convinced experts or the general public that this transformation has led to better quality or a more satisfied consumer, although no hard evidence of a significant decline in quality exists either. Physicians Elwood and Lundberg (1996: 5), two major observers of our current health system, assert that quality improvements will come about only when three conditions are met. First, there must be

> strong national standards that hold these plans accountable
> for the results they achieve—either in terms of clinical qual
> ity, improving the health of their enrolled population, or
> even satisfying the expectations of their enrollees. . . . Sec
> ond, then purchasers and consumers will be able to reward
> or punish plans based on quality. And third, when purchas
> ers and consumers have . . . the tools that allowed them to
> them to buy on quality, and if they could actually begin to
> use that power to shape the market.

Cost containment has made it possible to look away from health-care reform and even to consider ways of extending coverage to the uninsured. But managed care has also changed the nature of medical education and training and has raised questions about how to maintain quality during this era of lowered expenditures (and expectations). As we have seen, state legislatures, the president, and provider representatives are seeking to shape the future in a way that softens the excesses of managed care plans while sometimes grudgingly recognizing its advantages.

## REFERENCES

Eisenberg, J. M. 1996. "What went wrong with the Clinton Health Plan." *New England Journal of Medicine* 335 (August): 603. (July 8): A1, B6.

Elwood, P. M., and Lundberg, G. D. 1996. "Managed care: A work in progress." *Journal of the American Medical Association* (October 2). Pp. 1–9. http://www.ama-assn.og/ . . . ol_no_13ed6063x.htm

Freudenheim, M. 1996. "H.M.O.s are having trouble maintaining financial health." *New York Times* (June 19): D12.

Freudenheim, M. 1991. "In a stronghold for H.M.O.s, one possible future emerges." *New York Times* (September 2): 1, 28.

Gold, M. R., Hurley, R., Lake, T., Ensor, T., and Berenson, R. 1995. "A national survey of the arrangements managed-care plans make with physicians." *New England Journal of Medicine* 333 (December 21): 1678–1683.

Kerr, P. 1993. "Betting the farm on managed care." *New York Times* (June 27): Section 3: 1, 6.

Kilborn, P. T. 1996. "Tucson H.M.O.'s may offer model for Medicare's future." *New York Times* (March 26): A1, B11.

Meyerson, A. R. 1995. "Helping health insurers say no." *New York Times* (March 20): D1, D5.

Pear, R. 1996. "U.S. issues guidelines to help doctors form health networks." *New York Times* (August 29): A22.

Robinson, J. C. 1996. "Decline in hospital utilization and cost inflation under managed care in California." *Journal of the American Medical Association* 276 (October 2): 1060–1064.

Robinson, J. C., and Casalino, L. P. 1995. "The growth of medical groups paid through capitation in California." *New England Journal of Medicine* 333 (December 23): 1684–1687.

Roemer, M. I. 1973. "An ideal health care system for America." Pp. 77–93 in Anselm Strauss, ed., *Where Medicine Fails*. New Brunswick, N.J.: Transaction Books.

Rosenthal, E. 1996. "A pushy newcomer shakes up cancer treatment in New York." *New York Times* (September 8): 1, 44.

Winslow, R. 1995. "Employer group rethinks commitment to big HMOs." *Wall Street Journal* (July 2): B1, B4.

# 10
## Unresolved Issues Regarding Managed Care

The ultimate question is whether health care is a social good or a market commodity. If you believe health care is a commodity like food or automobiles or clothes, then that leads you down one road. If it's a social good like public health or clean air, you go down another.
—John C. Rother, AARP,
(Wines and Pear, 1996)

The 1996 presidential campaign seemed to avoid substantive discussion of health-care reform. After all, President Clinton had badly stubbed his toes early in his first term in his attempt to extend coverage to all Americans and bring down costs. His perception then had been that reform had to be done all at once in order for it to be effective. There were good reasons to pursue that direction if the goal was to attain savings and avoid cost-shifting as some types of care became more difficult to access. There was a grand design behind the Health Security Act, but unfortunately, Clinton and his advisors forgot to define his position in terms that ordinary Americans could understand. The result was that his political enemies successfully labeled his effort "government medicine."

In the 1996 presidential campaign, candidate Bob Dole tried to resurrect the specter of an octopus-like government strangling the citizenry with regulations once Bill Clinton was reelected. Calling Bill Clinton a liberal was similar to calling an opponent a communist 40 years ago; to define those terms was hard then, and it is hard now. But what many Americans responded to, then and now, was concern that they would lose something they had—access to good care. After all, only one out of eight Americans lacked health insurance.

The worry expressed about a bureaucratized system of health care was that the quality of care would decline. Little did anyone think that issues of quality would become a concern *without* health-care reform. Creeping capitalism in health care now became visible. As the editors of *Consumer Reports* concluded in October 1996, "managed care was a profit-driven, marketplace response to the health-care crisis." Some Americans began to feel that this driver was out of control.

But who put this driver in the driver's seat? Employers made HMOs the preferred way of purchasing health care for employees. True, the market forces that had been taking over health care during the 1990s did slow the growth of health-care costs for the under-65 population. Yet many complaints were being heard about the lack of concern being shown for consumer needs and the providers' judgment about how to practice competently in these closely watched and tightly controlled systems of care that were evolving.

The terms *dislocation* and *confusion* were being used to describe what was happening. Paul Elwood, who originally came up with the designation of health maintenance organization, began to label what he saw in 1996 "unmanaged competition." Even more frightening to ordinary people was that, whereas previously testing was routinely ordered to rule out serious and often life-threatening conditions, now conditions were routinely regarded as not worth the biopsy. In a few notorious incidents, overlooking a serious sign or symptom meant that treatment was started very late following the correct diagnosis made— often at a stage when medical care was made both difficult and more heroic than it need have been.

Some of these popular concerns were being noted in high places. Almost as if reconsidering a suitor who had been spurned for gauche behavior but had now stopped doing unpleasant things, the country seemed to find much to like about its young president. With Clinton's new sensitivity to problems that he could do something about and with much lowered expectations for change, he announced in early September 1996 that he would soon appoint a federal advisory commission to recommend ways of protecting consumers from some of the excesses of the system. Focusing on the changing health-care system and the quality of care, the newly formed National Commission on Health Care Quality would advise him on what legislation to pursue during his second term. The 20 panel members would be selected from the various stakeholders, including representatives of providers, insurers, labor, consumers, and business executives (Pear, 1996b).

While the president's initiative appeared worthwhile, who would get to serve on the commission? After all, the broad categories designated reveal little about which players would be named later. Some consumers have more at stake than others. Concern about access to care for the traditionally underserved (poor people) or those who feel that they will lose out under managed care would make this an important constituency when making appointments. At the time of the announcement, it was not clear whether consumer groups representing the disability community, a high-utilization population, would be named to the commission, or for that matter, representatives of Medicaid-eligible individuals.

The shift to managed care is only one of many recent social changes that have left many Americans anxious about whether their hard work and conforming behavior will provide them with the financial security needed to raise a family, develop personal interests, share a life with a partner, participate in community life, or do any of a thousand other worthwhile endeavors. The economic rewards for the lower middle class have continued to be ratcheted down, and health-care insurance coverage is just another of those things that can no longer be taken for granted. The global marketplace made Americans think hard about their future. Moreover, sacrifice for the next generation will not guarantee that one's progeny will live more affluent lives. Well-paid industrial jobs with benefits have been transformed into service-sector occupations without benefits or extremely scaled-down health plans.

In the past, Americans relied on the advice and counsel of their physicians. Even when most people were willing to say that the health-care system was in need of great reform, they were satisfied with their own health care. This contradiction was the reason why the health-care reform as outlined by the Clinton plan got such little support. Today concern has arisen that the basic trust we have had in physicians may be misplaced when they become part of a managed care organization. When physicians are perceived as benefiting financially from withholding services or not making referrals, then patients start to feel that they have less access under managed care than they had in the indemnity system. How can a health plan and the providers who work in them be seen as dependable if consumers begin to sense that the medical decision is no longer made according to medical criteria?

No doubt, indemnity insurance contributed to our current unacceptable expenditures on health care; yet there was still a sense that the doctor was working for you and not a corporation that would benefit from rationing care. Attorney Adam Yarmolinsky (1995: 602) describes this new anxiety over getting the best care; this fear has replaced confidence in the once secure payment and care system.

> In earlier years, after the potential cost of health care exceeded an individual patient's capacity to pay, patients for-

tunate enough to be insured treated their insurance policies
as open accounts. . . . Now, insured patients and physicians
are uncomfortably aware of a third party looking over their
shoulders, or worse still, threatening to withdraw its protection.

Despite this warning, some of the principles of managed care could
be adopted in any payment system. Few would argue with the premise
that managed care can lead to better care by eliminating treatments
that are both dangerous and ineffective, providing more proactive treatment, and establishing high standards for screening and early detection. Still, managers and physicians in HMOs are subject to cross
pressures: the need to provide care for the patient and not use up so
much in the way of resources so as to create less returns for investors
than anticipated or allow the nonprofit HMO to operate with a deficit.

The gatekeeping function of primary-care providers especially reveals some of the conflicts that occur in the payer–provider–patient
triangle. In the past, the physician was a trusted protector of the patient's interest and was not implicitly asked to balance the patient's
needs against those of the corporate entity that contracted for the physician's services. Some advocates for people with chronic illnesses or
disabilities argue that the various risk-sharing arrangements that
make the physician sensitive to using tests and making referrals to
specialists should not be allowed as a source of remuneration for physicians. Therefore, the gatekeeper should not be put in the position of
having to choose between obligations to patients and obligations to employer or payer for services. Financial incentives that encourage restraint in the delivery of services may mean that access to care is
limited arbitrarily.

Critics of managed care are especially concerned that unless protocols are closely followed, a serious condition will likely be misdiagnosed
as a minor illness or will be overlooked entirely. This increase in the
incidence of what is known as false negatives—the diagnosis of no disease being present when it actually is present—is a great worry. Several cases have led to litigation where precisely this type of error has
occurred in HMOs and where patients have died or suffered the serious
consequence of not receiving treatment for a treatable condition.

Reduced access to specialty care implies that precisely this kind of
error will increase when managed care becomes even more prevalent
than it is. Wherein past errors in medical diagnosis were likely to be
"false positive," or to identify disease states when they actually were
not there, the newer restraints on practice hardly encourage such outcomes. Litigation that follows misdiagnoses with harmful results involves both the physician and the plan.

Any health plan overtly enumerates its benefits and limits in detail when attempting to recruit individual consumers. Less explicit are the methods of restricting providers so that they cannot learn about how their access is limited. These limits can variously be harmless or full of consequences for consumers, and it is within their rights to know how their health plan's contracts with physicians impinges on their care and on information about their care.

Moreover, a patient sometimes has a rare condition that is best treated by an expert specialist who may not be a member of the plan. When a plan promises to provide all the medical care required, then even if patients come down with conditions that the HMO doctors are unfamiliar with, they still have to make state-of-the-art medical care available. Consumers want to know that a plan can actually say that it went the "extra mile" for a patient and delivered what was needed—not that it refused to pay for a consultation with a physician who is not a plan participant. This kind of preemptive refusal to seek the best medical care possible is similar to health insurers dropping enrollees who are making claims for covered services related to a catastrophic illness.

For a health plan to be of service to its subscribers, it must cover all medical contingencies, in much the same way that a fire department in a city provides coverage rights to the city's limits or borders. Sometimes neighboring departments cover for each other when an adjacent area is left vulnerable because resources are concentrated in a distant location. It would be unheard of to find out that the firefighters didn't answer an alarm because the location of the fire was inconvenient.

HMOs are not a public utility supplying all medical care needed. There is also sometimes the implicit restriction of access to needed care resulting from failure of knowing about all the options. Patients cannot make a clear decision when physicians restrict or withhold information. Most controversial are the previously discussed "gag clauses"—contract wording that forbids doctors from working for the patient in need. These restrictions interfere with the basic trust that must be established between doctor and patient. Marc A. Rodwin (1995: 605) raises some of the legal and ethical issues relating to who should protect the patient from lack of information.

> If managed-care organizations do not fully disclose their policies of limiting services, should physicians? Should physicians as fiduciaries also inform patients of medical options that managed-care organizations exclude? And should doctors inform patients of their own financial incentives to reduce services?

The quality of the health plan should include support for patients with regard to all the medical problems encountered, not just those approved treatments. With interventions the subject of evaluation, there is a need to determine whether they work and whether patients actually benefit from the procedures performed. This kind of inquiry seeks greater accountability. Thus, an attempt could be made to see if HMOs do a better job than fee-for-service indemnity coverage policies in keeping people well or in curing them.

In order to make such comparisons as well as comparisons between HMOs, data collection must include large enough samples so that age, level of severity of the disease, and other variables can be held constant. Employers who purchase group coverage through HMOs are becoming more and more concerned about quality benchmarks that go beyond signing up board-certified providers and high rates of immunization and screening (e.g., mammography).

The question remains, do these interventions make a difference? Although a cure rate is difficult to measure, it is possible to compare how well health plans are able to reduce cholesterol levels and hypertension, or prevent patients with diabetes from being hospitalized. These kinds of interventions have to do with management of serious chronic illness rather than simply followup of screening for chronic illness.

The development of such measures of accountability is particularly important as Congress encourages individuals eligible for Medicare to join HMOs. HMOs that specialize in this population will be under the closest scrutiny because the various encouragements of individuals over 65 to join HMOs will raise new questions about the quality of care under managed care. These new outcome measures are good for health care in general, but they come at a price. The shift to managed care has created more interest in quality measurement than in the past, but these health plans have had to spend more time and money justifying their existence. Health-service research has become a growth industry in the age of managed care.

In the past, this branch of research made some extraordinary discoveries, full of policy implications. One of the great discoveries of these investigators was that when complex procedures had to be done, there were differences in outcomes according to how frequently those interventions were performed. Thus, with regard to cardiac arterial bypass grafting, some surgeons did better than others, even when researchers controlled for the degree of severity of damage to the patients' heart and circulatory system that brought them in to face the knife.

Given the success of these busy surgeons, sick patients sought them out, and they developed a great deal of experience in treating this population. Experience seemed to count and be rewarded in the old fee-for-service system, and thoracic surgeons were admired who took on the most difficult cases. In the world of managed care, the successful surgeons may avoid the most critically ill because they increase the likelihood that they will have to spend more time with patients, order more tests, and prepare to operate.

How can our health-care system continue to reward the pursuit of excellence in medical practice and therefore encourage physicians and surgeons to gain experience working with the most difficult cases when the new managed care reward system is organized around risk avoidance?

Even strong advocates of free enterprise have noted that doctors are put in a peculiar position when the HMO pursues corporate profits. Colorado Republican State Representative Martha Kreutz has helped write legislation that would prevent HMOs from telling doctors that they cannot discuss such procedures as the treatment of certain cancers through bone marrow transplantation when the plan does not pay for it. While reluctant to increase government regulation of industry, Mrs. Kreutz admitted that it was not the way she wanted profit-making plans to work. "Yes, it's free enterprise. But I don't think most constituents understand that their health care is being weakened so a few people can make a lot of money" (Pear, 1996a: A12).

## ENDING THE CROSS-SUBSIDIZATION OF RESEARCH, TRAINING, AND CARE FOR THE UNINSURED

The penetration of markets by managed care organizations has weakened health care in another sense. Many medical tasks involve the continuous rebuilding of medicine's infrastructure through the creation of new knowledge and the renewal of human capital by exposing trainees or residents to the most difficult cases. In addition, these practical citadels of twentieth-century health care have often been the sources of charity care for those without insurance, including the homeless, undocumented aliens, or the near-poor who cannot qualify for Medicaid. The support of these activities was part of the "connective tissue" that held American society together, with the funding coming largely from indemnity insurance payments that generated a surplus for these nonprofit corporations to help provide for the commonweal.

To be sure, this is not the only source of support for research on patient care. Direct supports are available for clinical research in the United States through grants and contracts from various federal agencies such as the National Institutes of Health (NIH) and the Public Health Service, as well as through funds provided by the pharmaceutical industry's programs. Since 1988, funding from industry sources has for the first time eclipsed the research allocations made through the NIH. The for-profit sector outspent the NIH by 40 percent in 1994 (Burnett, 1996: 92). Even patients who are in experimental research protocols may receive reimbursement from insurance companies for the standard or routine part of their care in the course of complex clinical research. Through rigorous clinical research on *voluntary* human subjects who have given their informed consent, medical investigators learn about disease mechanisms and the types of interventions that are possible, and then they compare the relative effectiveness of different kinds of treatments.

Clinical research in academic medical centers (AMCs) has been built on the access of scientists, who were also medical doctors, to mechanisms for funding research activities with clinical revenues. When costs were not a major concern, research projects could be initiated and conducted so that the actual equipment and labor time could be buried in per diem costs. The easy relationship between payers and providers meant that some procedures were performed on patients or specimens were taken from them in order to advance knowledge rather than directly benefit the patient being treated. Today, HMOs may regard some patient-care services provided in hospitals as research-related and therefore as not representing a valid charge related to a hospital stay.

Some evidence also exists that when patients are enrolled in closed provider "networks," medical investigators may have reduced access to subjects for studies. This may occur because HMO contracts with hospitals forbid this kind of patient involvement in research activities. Participation in clinical research may be forbidden even when patients are truly passive participants in studies, as when their blood is drawn manifestly to determine the current state of their health, but specimens can also be used to learn something more about hematology. Moreover, the frequency of hospital admissions and the patients' lengths of stay are markedly lower for individuals in HMOs than for those with other kinds of coverage. While less hospitalization does save money, it also means an increase in the number of patients seen in ambulatory care.

Predictably, clinical research has already shifted to outpatient settings. The AMCs and medical schools are still concerned that their clinical research opportunities are going to be limited under this new set of market conditions, and so they are actively looking for other means of support. They are also searching out ways of being useful to the large HMOs that have not only captured many "covered lives" but also have accumulated surplus dollars that can be used to support clinical research. The excellent research facilities and talent available at AMCs and medical schools can also be complemented by the management and patient information systems found in large HMOs. With this knowledge, patients with conditions of interest to the investigators can be easily located and followed prospectively.

The problem for many physicians with an interest in clinical research is that they basically earned their livelihoods as clinicians, which allowed them to pursue their research interests. Protected time could be created for a clinical researcher who was generously rewarded for patient care so that a day a week could be devoted to these investigatory passions. In an AMC, this kind of activity was not regarded as unusual but was encouraged. Generally at an AMC, achieving high rank within an affiliated medical school was based mostly on scholarly publications in journals where the paper's merits were considered blindly by reviewers who were not privy to the authorship of the piece. In the promotion process in academe, much less attention is paid to patient care skills or teaching ability.

Now that fees-for-service are being deeply discounted, the specialist based in the AMC often has to spend five or more days to generate the amount of income that could earlier be counted on to be the result of four days of consultations. Time for research is less available than it once was. With the arrival of HMOs, the old assumptions no longer hold when clinical research has to be sustained, and a new arrangement, perhaps a new partnership, needs to be created. However, it will take some time to create this new compact.

In 1996 we saw only the beginning of interest in developing this new partnership. Mechanic and Dobson, writing in the health-policy journal *Health Affairs*, suggest that the time is right to

> begin to address key issues such as developing a framework for reimbursement and coverage decisions for patients in research protocols, a process for expediting coverage for high-priority clinical studies, parameters for sharing information, and training needs of clinical researchers and physicians. (1996: 88)

Just as fear has now arisen that research will suffer with this new payment system and way of organizing medical work, there is also concern that medical training will suffer. Traditionally, attending physicians devoted a portion of their day on site at hospitals and medical centers to teaching house staff (interns and residents). Primary-care physicians now working under capitation have far less control over their schedule than in the past. HMOs with high PCP/patient ratios have little flexibility in the working day, so there is little time to devote to teaching the next generation of physicians some of the finer points of care.

Specialists face a similar problem, although by contract they may not be expected to see so many patients per day. Again, the deep discounts from the standard fee that HMOs demand from participating physicians, in exchange for large numbers of referrals, means that doctors need to do more to reach the same level of remuneration that they had before the advent of managed care. While teaching in AMCs was donated or *pro bono* labor in the past, it still had value. These centers are seriously concerned about the shortfall in mentoring that was once assumed to come with the territory when a doctor received admitting privileges to a hospital.

Finally, as hospitals become tied into contracts with HMOs for inpatient care, they will have less surplus in their budgets to provide charity care for the uninsured. To their credit, hospitals and medical centers have been providing uncompensated care through surpluses derived from the per diem payments provided by third-party payers. Even with the shift to a prospective payment system for Medicare patients and subsequently for those with commercial insurance, an attempt was made to provide emergency care and sometimes hospital care for individuals without insurance. Federal law also prevented hospitals from receiving federal assistance if they turned away from Emergency Departments patients who had no insurance and could not afford to pay for services. As mentioned earlier, hospitals that had a disproportionate share of the burden of caring for the poor, the uninsured, and the elderly also received subsidies through provisions of Medicare and Medicaid.

During the last three decades, states became ingenious in developing mechanisms for collecting revenues from insurers to cross-subsidize medical care for those who were not eligible for Medicaid but could not afford to pay expensive medical bills and had no insurance. Some payers were excluded from this method of "taxing" third-party payers because they were self-insured. HMOs were also exempt from supporting these activities by contract with the hospital. Because the HMOs could guarantee hospitals extensive income in exchange for deep discounts, hospitals were willing to exempt them from supporting uncompensated care. Increasingly, hospitals found it harder and harder to sustain their charitable activities. Even government-financed programs have sought a way of living with managed care, and HMOs have to learn to see the mutual advantage of cooperating, even subsidizing, some functions that on first blush appear to be outside their scope of interest.

In 1992 there was a health-care crisis in the United States, and the president-elect vowed to do something about it. Health-care reform failed, but the well-capitalized growth of managed care accelerated the integration of services and restriction of access to hospitals and specialty care. HMOs have not done much to extend coverage to the uninsured, make health care more accessible than in the past, or eliminate financial woes for consumers. A 1995 national telephone survey of 3993 randomly selected respondents found that in the preceding year 31 percent had experienced one of three core problems associated with the publicly recognized health-care crisis of only a few years ago: an episode of being uninsured, a time when they did not get medical care that they thought they needed, a problem in paying medical bills (Donelan et al., 1996). Of course, some experienced all three problems. And most importantly, people in fair or poor health, people with serious chronic illnesses, and people with disabilities were disproportionately represented in all three problem areas. Vertical and horizontal integration may exist within HMOs, but both are certainly irrelevant for those who are unable to afford any insurance and cannot pay their medical bills. Perhaps they can receive help from state and local authorities.

## COORDINATION WITH PUBLIC HEALTH AGENCIES

A good society requires cooperation among all components of the health-care system. Putting compassion aside, HMOs and public health agencies share a common interest in limiting the spread of disease as a cost containment strategy. Yet, too often, HMO executives suggest that certain kinds of services are beyond their contractual responsibilities. The pattern in HMOs' purchases of services and in determining their charges is to avoid costs that do not reflect a service they absolutely must have and therefore must pay for. Similarly, physicians are required by federal law to perform certain public health and coordination activities with other agencies. Early intervention services to promote the stimulation of infants and toddlers who are suspected of having developmental lags require a moderate level of effort on the part of pediatricians to make sure that youngsters get evaluated. In addition, children with special health-care needs are entitled by law to specialty services as well as to care coordination as provided under the direction of each state's department of health.

The states' public health responsibilities tend to concentrate on prevention since avoidance of the spread of disease promotes a more productive population and less public and private resources will be spent on treatment. Therefore, state departments of health have mandated responsibility to protect the public from the spread of contagious diseases such as tuberculosis and sexually transmitted diseases. The means is through direct access to services for those who might avoid contact with medical providers because they cannot afford the price of the service. Family planning clinics have also been established to make their services available to the entire public, regardless of capacity to pay.

When states go into the business of converting Medicaid coverage to capitation, they may be paying twice for the same service. Managed care organizations are expected to provide access to care for contagious diseases as well as family planning as part of the array of services covered for one fixed fee. If a covered individual goes to a direct access program for one of these public health services, then the state needs to make sure that the health plan pays the direct access provider for the care extended.

Sometimes the plan will cover only the treatment of disease and will not cover other services that are provided during the course of a visit, as when someone is treated for a sexually transmitted disease but also gets family planning instruction or birth control devices. In the future, health plans and the state health departments must negotiate over who has what responsibilities in this package.

Health plans also collect a great deal of data on the health status of their enrollees. This information could be of great use to the public health authorities in assessing whether the Medicaid population requires additional essential services to stop the spread of communicable diseases or increase knowledge about family planning. A special report of that little known but important group, the Association of State and Territorial Health Officials (1995: 5), recommends that a coordinated effort be required to collect these data.

> Establish uniform reporting and tracking requirements by public and private organizations to provide surveillance information on public health priority areas. Costs of the state-wide early warning surveillance system should be borne by public and private sector health care organizations that benefit from the information.

All of this takes place in the presence of a shrinking government and fewer nonprofits in the delivery of health care and an expansion of the private for-profit sector. Private for-profit sector organizations often define their mission and accountability in a much more limited way than state or local governments or the voluntary sector. How will the public health of the community be maintained in the face of such enormous changes? Showstack and his colleagues (1996: 1071) have developed a guide that managed care systems can utilize in determining whether they are responsible contributors to the public common good. They suggest that each system must reflect on and "judge whether a managed care system is a responsible, accountable, and responsive contributor to the health of the community."

## ASSURING QUALITY WHERE IT THREATENS THE HMO'S ECONOMIC SUCCESS

What really counts when you go to the doctor? Most Americans would probably mention thoroughness, knowledge of the latest discoveries in medicine, and performance of appropriate preventive measures and screenings according to one's age. In addition, they would all talk about having contact with a doctor who cares about them as persons. Finally, since there are times when everyone needs contact with specialists, most would expect prompt referral for those services on an as needed basis.

The key then to good care is having someone you trust and a technically competent support system behind that person. Most of the current forms of evaluation that exist in the world of managed care are based on measuring what is easy to see—is the child up to date on immunizations? Now prevention is very important, but we need to know how these systems deal with deficiencies in the care of vulnerable people, particularly those with serious, chronic illnesses and disabilities.

Naturally, in a system where "less is more" this kind of evaluation component is vital. There is a tension in managed care that is based on having both to care for the patient but recognize that corporate survival, whether with or without profits, depends on not doing as much as could be done or would be done in another epoch. As physician-editors Marcia Angell and Jerome Kassirer (1996: 885) assert:

> The rapid growth of the quality industry underscores the essential paradox of the present health-care system. We have embraced a financing and delivery method that rewards doctors, sometimes quite directly, for doing less for their patients. Most doctors are now double agents—working for their patients but also for their companies.

The kinds of evaluations that health plans attempt to do are often shaped by organizational considerations related to marketing a product, largely to the benefits officers of large corporations. Standardized measures that include consumer satisfaction survey questions related to ease of access and courtesy extended are not vital concerns of people when they are sick. As novelist and literary critic Susan Sontag once noted when reflecting on her battle with cancer, when a person crosses over to that land of the sick, you hold a different identity and a different attitude. Then, as patients—not consumers—we are interested in the concern showed by our physicians, the appropriateness of the interventions that became part of the diagnostic and treatment plan, and the skill of the tasks performed. (As we get older and approach those years when serious, chronic illness is more likely, we begin to appreciate how hard it is to find the caring physician who knows what to do and can do it capably.)

With all the effort and money spent on developing the HEDIS system of evaluation and the CAHPS survey, little seems to be known about how to measure quality of care when complex medical interventions are undertaken. Given the concern about undertreatment in the managed care environment, particular attention must be paid to the critical omissions of interventions that would be universally regarded as appropriate. The constructors of HEDIS do not champion this measure of quality because there are too few cases of a particular condition in each plan to make meaningful statistical comparisons.

Part of the problem in measurement is that the easy-to-reach indicator does not always provide the best information about what is going on in a health plan. Just because the light is shining in this quadrant doesn't mean that what you really want to see will be found there. Purchasers may be happy with measures that provide a general assessment of whether the resources are deployed economically; this usually means a focus on the prevention and early detection or screening programs.

The demographics of the HMO should indicate that more than babies and young mothers are involved in the quality-of-care calculus. Perhaps we need to hear from others besides the measurement folk about what should count in writing a report card on a plan.

Doctors Elwood and Lundberg have developed some principles of accountability in a *Journal of the American Medical Association* editorial that go well beyond what is found in HEDIS or CAHPS (1996). Perhaps the following principles are idealistic, but they are laid out to provide guidance to a health-care system that is becoming increasingly given to "unmanaged competition."

- The quality measures must be powerful enough to provide direction to the American health system.

- The measures must anticipate the behavior changes they induce.

- Patient opinions should come first.

- It's time for outcomes accountability.

- The influence of health plans on the measures chosen should be minimized.

This editorial may be way out ahead of the American Medical Association; it is certainly out front of the American Association of Health Plans. But times are changing. Elwood and Lundberg are certainly preparing for the future.

These statements suggest that we should build a health-care system around the needs of patients and their providers, recognizing that quality programs not only keep people well but will attract sick people and that these programs should be rewarded for having that reputation. The growth of HMOs should not be resisted. Managed care is not the enemy of good medical care. What is needed is a way of putting patients and quality care first in our management decisions, our development of accountability, and our planning for the American health-care system's entry into the twenty-first century.

Some observers maintain that the basic trust between patients and physicians can be restored by recognizing their mutual interest, quite apart from the interest of health plans. Coming out of a sociologic tradition, Mechanic and Schlesinger (1996: 1693) argue that

> managed care plans rather than physicians should be required to disclose financial arrangements, that limits be placed on incentives that put physicians at financial risk, and that professional norms and public policies should encourage clear separation of interests of physicians from health plan organization and finance.

## WHO SHOULD CONTROL HMOs?

Clearly, most of us would not be interested in taking charge of such a huge operation. Still, input from the major players within the HMO might be very interesting. This would require a major transformation in the landscape. Still, there is support for the view that cooperation is both necessary and possible. Two advocates of this transformation, Steffie Woolhandler and David Himmelstein (1994: 266), suggest that a takeover of HMOs is required.

> We need control by patients and caregivers, not stockholders, managers and employers. We need medical integration, so that health care in communities is not carved up among ostensibly competing organizations, each avoiding financially unrewarding tasks and patients, and shunning community-wide cooperation.

Large HMOs have increased their reach through mergers (U.S. Healthcare and Aetna). Employers continue to tolerate questionable costs that are added when these managed care plans are marketed, generate profits for shareholders, and develop elaborate information systems. Still, privatization has not shrunk the system as much as it could be shrunk if these nonmedical expenses were eliminated. While the pace of inflation for health care has been slowed from what it was in the early 1990s, without overhead, profits, and other expenses, the inflation rate would have been reduced even more.

Profits are made when health-care expenditures are kept lower than the HMO's dollar intake. Known as the medical-loss ratio, this figure is used by profit-making HMOs to lure investors. With 65 percent of all HMOs being for-profit corporations, the battle to keep costs down focuses on what is spent on patient care rather than on what is spent on the business end of the HMO. The October 1996 *Consumer Reports* article on the financing of HMOs noted that readers who were members of for-profit HMOs were less satisfied with the quality of care received than those in nonprofit HMOs.

> The for-profit plans also had lower medical loss ratios. For-profit plans in our survey spent on average 79 cents of every dollar collected in premiums on medical care from 1992 to 1994, while the not-for-profits spent 91 cents or 15 percent more. (p. 33)

To make managed care work better, HMOs must be held responsible for what they do in a public way. Government oversight is necessary to ensure that patients get the care they need. State governments' current efforts to provide consumer protection, as reported in Chapter 8, is a step in the right direction.

One such program that is moving toward creating an independent grievance process recently became law in New Jersey. Though not mandatory, an independent utilization review organization (IURO) means that when the health plan internally rejects an appeal for authorization to receive a procedure, then it can be subject to an external review. Where the HMO's decision is not upheld, it has to provide clear justification for rejecting the independent panel's findings (State Health Watch, 1996: 3). The health plan bears the costs of the appeal process, and this factor will probably encourage HMOs to turn down fewer members' requests for costly procedures.

Finally, the Garden State, like many others, is introducing disclosure rules concerning compensation systems used for providers. The president of the state association of HMOs, Paul Langevin, argues in an interview (while turning incentive into a verb) that these reward systems are proprietary because they are "effective in incenting physicians to do the right thing without being so powerful an incentive as having them withhold care. And something that was so successful . . . is not something you would want to share with your competition" (*State Health Watch*, September, 1996, p. 3).

This comment gets to the heart of the matter—regardless of how for-profit health plans are organized. If a good system of care is available, maybe the equivalent of a cure or an immunization, and if it has the potential for helping many more people than are now subject to its reach, should not that approach be shared with all HMOs so that they can use it to save lives, promote well-being, or improve functioning? Would not keeping this a secret work against the mutually shared goal of providers and patients of supporting healthy outcomes? Surely, there is precedent for sharing a care system that is so beneficial to Americans that we could all gain from access to it.

The only way to make sure that this system of organizing health care is as good as it is claimed to be is to evaluate it and compare it against all competitors. This task may not be left to a voluntary program like NCQA but may have to be assigned to a government agency to make it compulsory.

The concept of managed care and HMOs, a uniquely American phenomenon, has arrived. Once condemned by the medical establishment as run by incompetent physicians, it has hit the covers of our weekly news magazines, gets minutes on magazine formats on television, has found a number of homes on the Internet (both in favor and against), and is likely to become the subject of a congressional investigation, maybe even before this book is in bound pages. It still has not convinced many who cannot afford insurance or have been turned away because of preexisting conditions that it is there for them.

Not only do HMOs not want to provide a low-cost product for the uninsured, but also former federal official, now a senior vice president at Prudential HealthCare, William Roper, has said flatly, "We are not in the business of giving away health services. The problem of the uninsured can only be solved by Government" (Consumer Reports, 1996: 35). Nor are they in the business of delivering medical services with low overhead costs, and they are not independent of the need to generate profits for shareholders. So while health care has rapidly changed in the direction of managed care, the question I raised in *Putting Health Care on the National Agenda* (1993) remains unanswered: How can we provide quality care for everyone at reasonable cost?

Managed care opens up some opportunities to save money by eliminating unnecessary services. But by introducing the need to cast a wide net and recruit millions to a plan, a lot of money is now spent on advertising. To assure buyers that the program is one of quality, millions are spent on accreditation, information gathering, and data analysis. To attract capital in order to continue to expand operations, profits must be shown, usually derived from reining in costs on medical services. To establish reserves to meet state insurance law requirements, additional revenues are required.

This dynamics takes place under conditions of fierce competition to gain contracts with employers. The larger the number of covered lives, the more cost effective is the effort to bring a prospective buyer into the plan. Lower unit costs means more profits. Indeed, virtually the same time, energy, and money are spent in sales if there are 1000 health-plan beneficiaries or 10,000.

Beneficiaries need to know what they are getting if they sign up with a health plan. This means not only what is covered by the plan but also how the providers are recruited, selected, compensated, and evaluated. In addition, it means how they are integrated into a health system that begins gently with routine office visits for well babies and ends with dramatic interventions such as heart transplants for old men. This must become public information because we are embarking on a new course in health-care delivery—one that was largely rejected by the public when the prospects of health-care reform were good. Americans did not want to choose a plan; they wanted to continue to choose their doctors.

Congressional Republicans strongly resisted reform, while the Clinton administration bungled it. During that diversion, the large employers bought into the HMO model of service because the price was right and their fringe-benefit costs could be contained, but choices of plans were substantially reduced. Only one out of three workers today has any choice of health plan at work.

As consumers of managed care, we need to have a bill of rights that protects us from poor plans, not just through a "report card" that rates them but through a system that guarantees the high quality of existing plans and eliminates those that don't come close to the quality of the top-rated HMOs. Those that flunk should be put out of business because they don't protect the consumer even when they make the purchaser feel that she is getting a good buy.

Profit making is good provided that the public can be assured that the product out there is not dangerous to their health or to the quality of their lives. Despite the bad language used to describe government bureaucracy today, few Americans assert that they want to give up environmental protections, the right to a free education for their children, public health, and safety standards for food and water as well as pharmaceuticals. Another protection might be added: A health-care system built around managed care that reserves part of the payment to providers for maintaining or improving the health of the lives that it covers, not just keeping the medical-loss ratio down. According to health-policy expert David Kindig, this kind of planning would, have to meld nonmedical factors in with medical interventions to improve health. It would also need to factor in the value of interventions as far as improving or maintaining the quality of life of those receiving assistance. These kinds of computations are far beyond the scope of this book, but readers should be aware that health-service researchers know a great deal about what interventions work to improve the quality of life. This is clearly an area of knowledge where government support and guidance through the Agency for Health Care Policy Research can help us to avoid supporting worthless interventions.

Government needs to perform some tasks so that we can get on with our lives. A division of labor promotes social solidarity and productivity, and also allows us to concentrate on what we do best. Regulation of health care, as part of that division of labor, is beyond the knowledge, ability, and motivation of ordinary citizens. But they can act best as citizens (and as consumers) when they have accurate information about how the institutions they depend on work.

If managed care is to improve on the old way of delivering health care, then it has to recognize the contributions of interested citizens, banding together to advocate for a bill of rights for health-care consumers in managed care settings. This protection cannot be written in stone but is subject to change as health-care delivery evolves. We may need the equivalent of a constitutional convention to write this document. Despite the enormity of this task, at least it will be the result of argument and debate among payers, providers, and patients, and not be settled in the board rooms of corporate America, by coalitions of small-business lobbies and insurance executives, or by the newly emerging congressional ramrods and ideologues.

Matters should not be left to manipulative groups who want the playing field to themselves, despite the transparent fact that they sincerely want to be rich. In the nineteenth century, European progressives proclaimed that medicine was too important to be left to physicians. And in the twenty-first century it will be too important to be left to corporate enterprise to shape as it sees fit.

## REFERENCES

Angell, M., and Kassirer, J. P. 1996. "Quality and the medical marketplace—following elephants." *New England Journal of Medicine* 335 (September 18): 883–885.

Association of State and Territorial Health Officials. 1995. "Special edition: Public health strategies for Medicaid managed care." *ASTHO Access Report*. Washington, D.C.: Association of State and Territorial Health Officials.

Burnett, D. A. 1996. "Evolving market will change clinical research." *Health Affairs* 15 (Fall): 90–93.

Consumer Reports. 1996. "Can HMOs help solve the health-care crisis?" *Consumer Reports* (October): 28–33.

Donelan, K., Blendon, R. J., Hill, C. A., Hoffman, C., Rowland, D., Frankel, M., and Altman, D. 1996. "Whatever happened to the health insurance crisis in the United States? Voices from a national survey." *Journal of the American Medical Association* 276 (October 23/30): 1346–1350.

Elwood, P. M., and Lundberg, G. D. 1996. "Managed care: A work in progress." *Journal of the American Medical Association* 276 (October 2): 1083–1086. .ol_276/no_13ed6063x.htm

Mechanic, R., and Dobson, A. 1996. "The impact of managed care on clinical research: A preliminary investigation." *Health Affairs* 15 (Fall): 72–89.

Mechanic, D., and Schlesinger, M. 1996. "The impact of managed care on patients' trust in medical care and their physicians." *Journal of the American Medical Association* 275 (June 5): 1693–1697.

Pear, R. 1996a. "Laws won't let H.M.O.'s tell doctors what to say: 16 states give patients right to be informed." *New York Times* (September 17): A12.

Pear, R. 1996b. "Clinton to name health-care panel, with eye on second term." *New York Times* (September 6): A20.

Rodwin, M. A. 1995. "Conflicts in Managed Care." *New England Journal of Medicine* 332 (March 2): 604–607.

Showstack, J., Lurie, N., Leatherman, S., Fisher, E., and Inui, T. 1996. "Health of the public: The private-sector challenge." *Journal of the American Medical Association* 276 (October 2): 1071–1074.

State Health Watch. 1996. "NJ officials stand by proposed HMO rules for external appeal and reporting of compensation." *State Health Watch* (September): 3, 11.

Wines, M., and Pear, R. 1996. "President finds benefits in defeat on health care." *New York Times* (July 30): B8.

Woolhandler, S., and Himmelstein, D. U. 1994. "Galloping toward oligopoly: Giant H.M.O. 'A' or giant H.M.O. 'B'?" *The Nation* (September 19): 265–268.

Yarmolinsky, A. 1995. "Supporting the patient." *New England Journal of Medicine* 332 (March 2): 602–603.

# Bibliographical Essay

There are few books on managed care or health maintenance organizations, although in the next few years we will probably see them rival self-help books in number. The study of the Kaiser-Permanente Northwest Region consumers and providers by Donald K. Freeborn and Clyde R. Pope—*Promise and Performance in Managed Care* (1994)—provides a look inside a contemporary prepaid group practice. Less researched are the more rapidly growing network and independent practice association models.

The backdrop of my book is the recent effort to reform our health-care system. There is now a growing literature on why the Clinton health-care reform effort failed. While this subject is touched on briefly here, mainly to set the stage for an analysis of the origins, development, and consequences of managed care, the works of Paul Starr and Theda Skocpol are mentioned often as important analyses.

I have depended more on Haynes Johnson and David Broder's *The System* in order to understand the external forces that lined up against reform and the internal problems faced by the often-fractious Democratic party. Written by two *Washington Post* columnists and Public Broadcasting commentators, this popular work is special because some chapters are based on extended interviews with the major players in reform, including President Clinton, never one to shy away from commenting on his failures as well as his successes.

There are also some more recondite works on the failure of reform that explain not only what went wrong but also why the numbers did not add up. *The Problem That Won't Go Away: Reforming U.S. Health Care Financing*, edited by Henry J. Aaron of the Brookings Institution, attempts to answer the questions: Why did the Clinton health-care reform campaign fail? Who were the killers? The contributors suggest that part of the answers rest with a targeted fear campaign aimed at a public that was not terribly well informed about how health care is paid for and why coverage for all is a good idea. Since educating the public never took place, the attacks on the Health Security Act were never answered. The fear of more taxes was raised by the admirable Clinton commitment to cover the uninsured by either public or private insurance plans, whether through borrowing money and increasing the deficit, transferring income from the affluent to the subaffluent, or enforcing an employer mandate that says it is the obligation of all, not just big employers, to help pay for the group coverage created for their employees. Fearmongers in the Republican party used the emphasis on managed care as an extension of government to pull support away from the proposed Health Security Act. In the end, the American public, 85 percent of whom were insured, decided to trust the devil they knew rather than the one they didn't know.

There are several additional and sophisticated parts to the scholarly *The Problem That Won't Go Away*. Part II deals with what kinds of information are needed to estimate the effects of reform, handled adroitly by Linda Bilheimer and Robert Reischauer, former director of the Congressional Budget Office. This is followed by a rather elegant argument in Part III for market-based reform—managed competition and the use of purchasing alliances—by Alain C. Enthoven and Sara J. Singer and a discussion of where antitrust enforcement fits into future reforms. Finally, Part IV provides what might be called a roundup of the usual speakers from diverse political perspectives, wherein they discuss incremental reform, including steps toward universal coverage, the conservative agenda and medical savings accounts, cost cutting, and that 1000-pound gorilla on our backs—Medicare's disproportionate growth as we approach the end of the millennium. Missing from this worthwhile effort is an advocate for a single-payer approach to financing, which is perhaps the only way we can provide good health care for everyone at reasonable cost.

Because little has been published on managed care in monographic or extended essay form, I was dependent on many articles and editorials from medical and health-policy journals such as the *New England Journal of Medicine, Journal of the American Medical Association*, and *Health Affairs*. In particular, the continuously fine work on the changing financing of the health-care system by John K. Iglehart in the *New England Journal of Medicine* stands out. The national press, sometimes described as elitist, was helpful in dealing with late-breaking policy questions, details of the business end of health maintenance organizations, and consumer responses to managed care. My home-delivered *New York Times* often made me late for work as I attempted to read lengthy articles about our changing health-care system. I am especially indebted to the excellent analysis and reporting by Robert Pear and Milton Freudenheim. I read less systematically the *Washington Post* and the *Wall Street Journal*, two other papers that keep up with the revolution in managed care. *Consumer Reports* has been involved in analyzing the growth of managed care, the response of its readership, and the way to make managed care work, for the past 15 years. The weekly news and business magazines, in their consumer-friendly ways, also featured stories about the best and worst in HMOs. Finally, timely and impartial studies on controversial aspects of health care are prepared by the Congressional Budget Office and the United States Government Accounting Office.

Medicaid managed care does not get much attention in the weekly news magazines because, unfortunately, its beneficiaries are not big readers. A few monographs have been published on Medicaid managed care, including J. L. Buchanan et al.'s 1992 work—*Cost and Use of Capitated Medical Services: Evaluation of the Program for Prepaid Managed Health Care*. There is also the Robert Hurley and others 1992 monograph, *Managed Care in Medicaid: Lessons for Policy and Program Design*, and Diane Rowland and others' Kaiser Commission book, *Medicaid and Managed Care: Lessons from the Literature* (1995). Many unpublished works, (cited in Chapter 3) can be acquired by writing to the state agencies or national voluntary associations that produced them.

A similar bibliographic pattern appears in Chapter 4, which contains a mix of references to medical journals, health-services journals, and unpublished works. There is the one outstanding contemporary work on how to improve our health-care delivery, by Berwick, Godfrey, and Roessner, *Curing Health Care: New Strategies for Quality Improvement* (1990), cited in Chapter 5. Stewart and Ware introduce the concept of medical outcomes and how to study them in their 1992 *Measuring Functioning and Well-Being*.

Consumer satisfaction is reported in the national press, in *Consumer Reports*, and in a major ongoing contemporary study by the Commonwealth Fund. Note that the Commonwealth Fund study can be found on the World Wide Web, along with numerous other sources cited in *Managed Care: Made in America*. Legislative efforts to protect consumers and providers are documented in recent issues of *State Health Watch: The Newsletter of State Health Care Reform*.

The subject of professional autonomy is most thoroughly investigated by Bradford Gray in *The Profit Motive and Patient Care: The Changing Accountability of Doctors and Hospitals* (1991). The American Medical Association's 1996 study, *Medical Groups in the US: A Survey of Prac-*

*tice Characteristics*, is useful for learning how medical practice is changing and Berenson, Hastings, and Kopit's chapter on the legal framework for effective competition appears in the authoritative 1996 anthology by Stuart Altman and Uwe Reinhardt, *Strategic Choices for a Changing Health Care System*. Organizational and professional integration is also discussed in *Strategic Choices*. This work will be quoted frequently in the coming years when policy experts write about the future of health care.

# Index

## About the Author

ARNOLD BIRENBAUM, a health-care policy analyst, medical sociologist, and health services researcher, is Professor of Pediatrics at Albert Einstein College of Medicine and Associate Director of the University Affiliated Program for People with Developmental Disabilities, Rose F. Kennedy Center. He has authored or edited eleven earlier books and monographs, including *Putting Health Care on the National Agenda* (Praeger, 1995).